Rekindle your desire in 7 steps

A quick and effective strategy to improve your sexual desire

MYRIAM RIBES

Rekindle
Copyright © 2023 Myriam Ribes

All rights reserved.
No part of this book may be reproduced, or stored in a retrieval system, or transmitted in any form or by any means, electronic, mechanical, photocopying,recording, or otherwise, without express written permission of the publisher.

Cover design by: Txema Coll
Book Translation: Carlota Fluxà
Proofreading and editorial review: Carlota Fluxà and Anna Pérez
Layout design: Fabián Vázquez: www.fabianvazquez.net
ISBN: 9798861699792

Legal deposit number: ME - 778/2023

INTRODUCTION

Hi! I'm delighted you're here, and I'm thrilled that you are interested in your health. No, don't double-check the title of this book; you're not mistaken. It is indeed called "Rekindle Your Desire" and that's exactly what we're going to work on. But I assure you that everything you do to reawaken your desire will also enhance your health, because sexual well-being is one of the most important components of your health and overall quality of life.

SEX IS GOOD

Yes, good sex improves your health; this has been scientifically proven. Experiencing sexuality in a healthy and positive way combats stress, insomnia and chronic pain, makes us happier and more sociable, and also appears to reduce the incidence of many chronic diseases like cardiovascular disorders and cancer.

SEX IS HEALTHY

This is why I always find it hard to believe that there are people, institutions and governments that still assert that sexuality is not important. Even the World Health Organization (WHO) affirms that it is a central aspect of human life, and has established costly strategies and resources to improve the sexual lives of all people. That's because sexual health is vital, and because we all have the right to experience full sexuality -- consciously and free from prejudice!

WE HAVE THE RIGHT TO SEX WITH SENSE AND WITHOUT JUDGMENT

We all care about sex. No matter what you might say and whatever they might say, I assure you that sex is always a matter of interest. I'll share a personal story that proves it...

A few years ago, I set up my private practice next to a well-known ophthalmology center. I adore the owner, Dr. Concha Valero, an exceptional woman. She helped me in every way she could. Working near the Valero-Bosch family is a real privilege.

On the buzzer panel in the foyer, the button for my office was located just beside theirs. The one for the Ophthalmology Center read "Doctor's Office" so I decided to put my name on mine. I wrote my last name in big capital letters, so there would be no mistaking my buzzer: RIBES. But when I tested it, the buzzer didn't make any noise. I found that within the intercom box in my office, the wires were ripped out. I thought this was odd, but I reconnected them. When I tried it again, it rang – my little buzzer was working. I was so excited! I was ready to start seeing patients in my new practice. That very afternoon I would make my debut.

I soon understood why the previous tenant had pulled apart the wires. I became rather tempted to do the same myself. Even though I only had two appointments that afternoon, I had to answer the buzzer ten times. Ten! And all those calls were from people going to the other office, where I promise there is no one named Ribes. I suspected that perhaps the difficulty in distinguishing the buttons was visual -- let's not forget that they were going to an ophthalmology center. I spoke with Concha, and we decided to set up a separate intercom. And so we did. It looked beautiful. It was set apart from the other one, right beside my nameplate. This way nobody would mistake the two buzzers again.

The next afternoon... twenty people rang the wrong doorbell! I couldn't believe it. The new intercom attracted so much attention that people only noticed mine. I didn't know what to do! I tried GYNECOLOGIST in giant letters, but still no change. I decorated the whole intercom with pink hearts. But there were never less than fifteen calls each afternoon. No one actually read what the sign said. They saw something new and buzzed it. I was getting desperate.

Suddenly, I had an idea. I removed the hearts, removed GYNECOLOGIST, removed my name, and just put in capital letters: SEXOLOGIST.

That afternoon, only one person buzzed and when I opened the door, she was already fleeing in terror toward the other office, stammering a thousand apologies for having rung the wrong button.

"I didn't mean to call, I'm sorry, excuse me, I made a mistake, I was going the other way...," she said.

The word SEXOLOGIST was the solution. Including the word SEX finally made people really scrutinize the sign on the buzzer. But not only did it attract their attention, it also scared them.

SEX ATTRACTS OUR ATTENTION, BUT IT SCARES US

Yes, it scares us. And the fact is, that despite it being something so important, we don't seem to enjoy very good sexual health, or at least not the way we wish. Scientific studies report a very high incidence of sexual problems: 40% sexual dysfunction in women and 30% in men. More than a third of the population – that's a lot!

THE PREVALENCE OF SEXUAL PROBLEMS IS VERY HIGH

The most common consultation, the one that is most frequently asked about in sexology clinics, is the loss of desire, especially for couples who have been together a long time.

"Myriam, listen, I just want you to know that I'm only here because of my partner. For me, not having a sexual appetite is not a problem; I could live perfectly well without sex."

"I'm here to see if you can maybe give me something to make me want to have sex again, because after saying 'no' so many times, he'll leave me for another woman and not care about me anymore."

"I already do it without any desire to avoid the fuss and the unpleasant faces, but if I can, I wriggle out of it. If I can, I just slip away, try to avoid it or pretend I'm asleep."

"The worst thing is that I don't even touch him or kiss him goodnight anymore, in case he gets aroused and wants more than that."

Does this sound familiar? Could you have said it yourself?

Life as a couple is a challenge from Day One: the problems of living together, the fatigue of everyday life, the worries of work, life changes, family... And although good sex is no guarantee of a good relationship, it's clear that when it's not working, it ends up making a relationship worse. Sex is important for a couple: it connects us, strengthens us, and reconciles us.

We know that there are people who can live entirely without sex, who don't miss it if it's not a part of their life. Every person is different, and has different needs. But this book is not intended for them. I wrote Rekindle Your Desire thinking of people like you, who do miss it and want to change.

Do you worry about what is happening to you? Do you miss your sexual desire? Would you like to get it back? There are many important areas in life, but if love and sex aren't working, it can seem that nothing else does either. On the other hand, when they do work, everything seems possible. Imagine for a moment that with just a few changes in your routines you could once again feel that spark you miss so much. Imagine that you could even keep it forever.

Isn't it worth a try?

I strongly believe that everything happens for a reason and that things come when the time is right. My life has not been easy, although many people are surprised when I tell them that. It must be because they consider that my calm and friendly demeanor gives no hint of a difficult existence. But really, my life got off to a pretty bad start. My childhood was very tough and my adolescence even worse. And I confess that on several occasions I thought about ending it all and stopping all the suffering. Thank goodness I didn't, because when I least expected it, everything changed. My angels, my sweethearts appeared. They supported me, they healed me, and little by little they taught me how wonderful love is. Today I feel immensely happy. I am proud of and grateful for all the good things in my life, but I'm also grateful for all the bad that has happened to me, because it's made me the way I am and has led me directly to where I am: with the best people in the world.

That is why I know that everything is possible. That it's possible to overcome suffering and grow. That even the most toxic things can be recycled and transformed into works of art. And that is also why I have the urge to write. And I would like to share everything I've learned as a professional and as a person, to be able to give you the love that life has given me.

I have devised this book for you, whomever you are and wherever you are from. I want it to be useful to you whether you feel like a woman, a man, or any combination in the infinite universe of gender. I don't care about how you dress, whether you have a penis, a vulva, or both, what you like or what turns you on. I always write for you. And though I write from a feminine perspective, I do not intend to exclude or discriminate against anyone. It's simply a way of speaking: mine. Whoever you are and however you look, however you feel, I invite you to include yourself in the femininity that I feel: inclusive, plural and diverse.

I HOPE YOU LIKE IT

I WANT YOU TO ENJOY IT

I WANT TO HELP YOU REGAIN YOUR PASSION

To do so, I propose you try a strategy based on seven steps, similar to what I use in my practice, workshops, and courses.

In each step we will explore a theme, and I will propose a series of reflections and exercises. Step by step, chapter by chapter, you will make changes that work together to achieve your goal. I recommend you read one chapter each week, and during those seven days integrate everything that you've learned, remembered, and re-examined in that chapter. But you could also read the entire book in one sitting, then reread it slowly while doing the exercises. Or if you wish, follow a different order and manage the time as it works for you. Feel free to choose whatever suits you best. It is YOU, always YOU, who has the key to success. I have only given you a few clues for finding the key in the pages of this book.

DO YOU FEEL LIKE A PLEASURE RIDE TOWARDS DESIRE?

ARE YOU IN?

"Each one gives what he receives
And then receives what he gives
Nothing is simpler
There is no other rule
Nothing is lost
*Everything is transformed"**

JORGE DREXLER: Todo se transforma

https://www.youtube.com/watch?v=QfhEKpFiepM

*Suggested translation from the original lyrics

ACKNOWLEDGMENTS

No one shines alone. People are social creatures, and we grow by supporting one another. The excellence of our companions brings out the best within ourselves. That's why it's inevitable that I am and will be HUGE, because I have the most wonderful people by my side. Thank you. Eternal eons of gratitude for always sticking with me, even if I can't name each and every one of you. This book would not exist without you.

ϴ To Txema, the love of my life, for loving and supporting me so much.

ϴ To Mar and Biel, my miracles, my pride and my source of eternal gratitude.

ϴ To my twin sister Marisa, because for us, it's not a matter of blood but love, and it's impossible to have more than we do.

ϴ To Socorrito and Tino, my first teachers, for giving me life -- and the claws to hold on to it.

ϴ To Abe, the balm of my childhood, for his unconditional and boundless love.

ϴ To Anna, Carol, Jaime and Toni, my adventure partners, with whom I hope to travel year after year and life after life.

- To my family in Menorca, Cantabria, and in other corners of the earth. Thank you for always being family regardless of blood or distance.

- To my professional friends and colleagues. I have you all in mind: my girls from the CSP; my reunited XII class; my colleagues from Girona, from the capital, and from the volcanoes; my Diatros girls; my tribe of masters' students; and very specially my colleagues at the Mateu Orfila Hospital, who have supported me so much through my cataclysms. The pandemic has brought us closer than ever. I love you all so dearly.

- To all of you I call friends the world over; my saviors, my caregivers, my cared-for, and all who have encouraged me to write.

- To Fabián and Albert. I promise you, I will get to fiction too.

- To Vishen Lakhiani and his MindValley for waking me up. To Verónica and Florencia Andrés for giving me back my confidence.

- To Ana Nieto, for providing me with the tools and faith to succeed with my book as she does with hers.

- To all the people who work their fingers to the bone to make the world a better place.

- To the Mediterranean sea and land, my eternal destination.

- To my angels, whose wings fill with love every day of my life.

FOREWORD

I met my dear friend and sister Myriam ("Myri") Ribes in 2010 during the first promotion of the Clinical Sexuality Masters' Degree taught in Madrid by the UNED. When I entered the room, she was already seated. As we introduced ourselves, I heard her sweet shy voice for the first time.

"Hello, I am an OB/GYN and I come from Menorca."

At the time, I knew very little about Menorca, and I had no idea that years later, we would be working together in Mahón. What a gift life has given us.

When the Masters' was completed, its director, Andrés López de La Llave, invited us to participate in the Latin American Congress of Sexology and Sex Education. And that is when our story of love and desire began. Desire to love and support each other always. Desire to help each other achieve our goals and wishes.

And Myri's desire has always been...to write, to sit and watch the sea...and to write.

"I'm happy doing it, the hours fly by like seconds. This is what I really want to do: write."

She always said so, and this book, her first book, is full of enthusiasm and love. It's really how Myri does everything in life. She puts her commitment, her desire, and her love into everything she does. She is a great communicator because she communicates with presence, respect, modesty and affection. She makes difficult things easy and manages to make you feel comfortable, which is very important, especially in this case, as we are talking about SEX and DESIRE.

I know that in this book you will find many answers and skills to improve your desire and your sexual health. It is easy, enjoyable, and generates a lot of curiosity. I am sure it will be the first of many...

I hope you enjoy it as much as I did.

Thank you Myri, sister dear.

Marisa García Roso

All you need is LOVE

ALL YOU NEED IS LOVE

Of course you know this Beatles song. You must have heard the chorus a thousand times in your life. It's often played at weddings, in rom-coms, Internet videos, and as background music for lots of TikToks. During the 2020 confinement in Spain due to the COVID pandemic, it was played many afternoons, between rounds of applause for health care workers, protests, and all the multimedia manifestations that this strange era gave us.

Love is all you need

The Beatles premiered the song on the BBC's Our World program on June 25th, 1967. It was the first globally broadcast song on satellite television, and was seen live by over 700 million people in 30 different countries. All You Need is Love is considered one of the band's most famous songs; according to Rolling Stone magazine it is one of the 500 greatest songs of all time, and is considered a universal hymn of love and peace.

There's nothing you can do that can't be done

Since it's one of my favorite Beatles songs, when I found out that Moments a Cor, the gospel choir I sing in, was going to add it to its repertoire, I begged the director to sing the solo.

"Elsa, can I do it? I freaking love that song."

Elsa Perches is as sincere as she is a good director. She looked at me in amazement.

"You? Do you want to do the solo?"

She was surprised, and that made sense. I don't have the best voice, and I don't have the best stage presence. In fact, I'm scared to death and shy whenever I sing alone. I even feel embarrassed to be overheard while singing in the shower.

"Yeah, well... only if you're ok with it. It's just that... this is my song."

"Well, I'm sorry, Myriam, but I already have a soloist assigned to it. But I'll put you down as understudy, if that's OK."

"Super! That's great. Thank you very much!"

I sighed and thought it might also be better not to do it. When I sing along with the group I'm not afraid or nervous, so I'd be able to enjoy the song more. My song. Performing the solo, singing by myself, would have been terrifying. Although it could also have been mind-blowing. I imagined myself in the theatre, singing with my backing vocalists, driving the audience crazy, closing my eyes with the mic in my hand, and Lennon's spirit fluttering around me among rainbows and pink elephants. I would become Lennon's prophet on Earth.

Nothing you can sing that can't be sung

At the next choir rehearsal, Elsa approached me.

"Myriam, the soloist in All You Need told me she can't do the solo: you'll do it"

I jumped for joy. I was going to sing my song! All the other women congratulated me, and I felt very lucky. I went home smiling as if I were floating on a cloud. I had done it. But my bliss didn't last long before I was struck by terrible stage fright. And I came to my senses: although I love music, I was not born with a talent for musical interpretation. What was I going to do? I didn't want to make a fool of myself! I was about to call Elsa to tell her I was quitting, but suddenly, looking at the score, the words of the song possessed me.

And with it John Lennon, his rainbows and as many pink elephants as one can see without taking acid.

It's easy: all you need is love

It was easy! All I needed was love. LOVE. Love for me, for the song, for what I was doing, for my choir sisters, my director, the audience. And John Lennon. I only had to put love into it. That was the magic ingredient.

And I did: I lovingly rehearsed every day, lovingly learnt the lyrics, practiced my pronunciation with the utmost British love, I worked hard with love, sweat and tears, and finally, I put all that LOVE on stage. And the truth is, it didn't turn out too badly.

Nowhere you can be that isn't where you're meant to be

"Hey, Myriam. Not bad at all, not bad at all."

"Hey girl, where did you hide that voice? You always sing so softly!"

"Myriiiiiiiii. You sounded like a real rock star!"

"Oh Myriam, I was moved by the passion you put into it. I got goose bumps."

My choir sisters love me so much that they never say anything bad to me. They are that wonderful. But I had also noticed a different energy, a gush of excitement and passion overflowing from my body.

I repeated the solo a few times: in the theatre and at the weddings of two couples I love dearly. These might not have been the best performances of Moments a Cor, but they were very worthy and moving. I feel proud to have sung it and to have demonstrated the meaning of my favorite song with my own interpretation.

And, as you may have guessed, All You Need is Love is not only a hippie symbol of universal love, it is my anthem -- my way of seeing things, and my motto. Because if you put love into what you do, you'll make even the tiniest voice shine.

Love, love, love

Why is it that some people cook the same recipe better than others? Why do some people's orchids bloom year after year and others wither and die?

Life rewarded me with the best mother-in-law anyone could ever wish for. Esperanza was a wise, confident woman, ahead of her time, and brimming with love and wisdom. With all the things she taught me, I could write ten books like this one. She was good at everything, but she had one gift I truly envied: she was able to bring plants back to life. She used to take the orchids that I had dying at home and after a couple of day at hers, they looked like new.

"Geez... what's your secret? I've never been good with plants."

She laughed and shook her head.

"That's because you don't love them enough, Myriam. Plants just want your love and your time."

"But I do love them! Especially orchids."

"But you don't love them enough. You have other priorities that take over."

She was right. I didn't devote enough love to them because my priorities were elsewhere, but my mother-in-law's heart was so big that her yard was like a verdant orchard.

IF YOU PUT YOUR HEART INTO IT, YOU ALWAYS WIN

If you're reading this book, it's because you're looking for passion and you don't know how to find it. I hope you catch some of the passion that I have put into it, and invest it into what you want. I always put love into what I do (except for plants, I'm afraid.) I have embarked on this great health project with all my love. Because I am firmly convinced that if you are passionate about it and you work at it, you can overcome any obstacle. Bring passion, love and desire into your life, and you will be able to achieve almost anything you want. Maybe you'll even be able to revive drooping orchids.

WHAT IS DESIRE?

The other two, slight air and purging fire,
Are both with thee, wherever I abide;
The first my thought, the other my desire,
These present-absent with swift motion slide.
For when these quicker elements are gone
In tender embassy of love to thee,
My life, being made of four, with two alone
Sinks down to death, oppressed with melancholy;
Until life's composition be recured
By those swift messengers return'd from thee,
Who even but now come back again, assured
Of thy fair health, recounting it to me:
This told, I joy; but then no longer glad,
I send them back again and straight grow sad.

WILLIAM SHAKESPEARE: SONNET XLV

Desire is a beautiful word that refers to the energy that drives us to our yearnings, dreams and ambitions. When we talk about sexual desire, or libido, this is the impulse that motivates us to enjoy our sexuality, to be capable of affective intimacy, to maintain satisfying sexual relationships, and to experience pleasure.

We have the idea that desire is an automatic reflex, that it arises without thinking, that it is something that unexpectedly captivates us and ignites us like a match. And indeed, it can be extremely intense, especially in the early stages of a relationship. But desire is never truly irrepressible or irresistible, and it never justifies an inappropriate or criminal action. It is not desire that is irrational, but the behavior of some people.

Desire is the result of a complex interaction between sensory and psychological stimuli, emotional predisposition, and a wide number and variety of neurohormones. Broadly speaking, there are two different types of desire: active and reactive.

Active desire

This is the best known type of desire and the one that resides in our collective imagination. It is fiery and spontaneous, that intense impulse that moves you to seek sex and doesn't need stimuli to provoke it. It is typical of the beginning stages of a relationship, and it diminishes over time.

Reactive desire

This is intelligent desire; it is rational and voluntary. It is activated by concrete stimuli that awaken the libido, and the stimulus can be different for every person: caressing, gazing, speaking... This desire can persist and grow over time. It is a grateful desire that responds to whoever invests in it. Remember when we talked about putting love into things? Well, this is a good example: reactive desire is intelligent and it is built over time. It can be maintained throughout all stages of a relationship. In some relationships, desire may never have been spontaneous, and may have been built up intelligently from the start.

There is a logical parallel between these two types of desire and the phase of the relationship in which they occur. Active desire is characteristic of the early stages of a relationship, when one is falling in love, and reactive desire is typical of relationships that have evolved over a longer period of time, where conscious or mature love predominate.

Falling in love

It is that time when you live for and with your object of desire, and your desire is totally active. During this phase, which typically lasts from three months to three years, an unreal, perfect, and tailor-made image of the loved one is created, so wonderful that nothing makes sense without them.

This is all due to a cascade of intense neurohormonal changes, because love is pure biochemistry: the saying "you and I have chemistry" is absolutely true.

The first protagonists of this phase could be pheromones—chemicals that many animal species secrete and release into the environment with communicative and, above all, reproductive purposes.

Despite the efforts of the fragrance industry, it has not yet been proven that chemical compounds such as androstadienone and estratetraenol, which are sold as human pheromones, increase the level of desirability of their wearer to others. What is quite possible is that there are volatile chemicals, whether they are called pheromones or not, that allow us to perceive certain qualities in those who secrete them. These qualities could foster attraction between people with different genetic and immune systems, thereby enhancing the survival of the species.

Did you know that in New York City a new form of matchmaking called "pheromone parties" was introduced? It has already been imported by several European capitals. You're required to bring a T-shirt that you've slept in for three nights in a row. Each T-shirt is assigned a number, and participants choose their date for the night by the scent of the shirt.

Sexual attraction, whether or not it is mediated by pheromones, promotes eroticism and activates the secretion of endogenous substances such as testosterone, adrenaline and noradrenaline. The well-being, energy, and biochemical optimism that these substances generate make us fall in love, and they activate new brain areas and new substances. If we then add dopamine, serotonin and phenylethylamine, the resulting cocktail produces the well-known biological and emotional changes that characterize the infatuation phase:

tachycardia, nervousness, insomnia, the familiar butterflies in the stomach, loss of appetite, euphoric moments alternating with immense sadness when the partner is absent, increased sexual desire, obsessive thinking, loss of objectivity, and a distorted perception of reality.

The Spanish philosopher Ortega y Gasset was absolutely right when he said that being in love is a state of transient mental alienation, because due to these changes you become numb, and addicted to your partner.

- Your perception of reality is altered and you only see the positive aspects of your partner and your relationship. "Love is blind"
- Obsessive and fixated thinking about the loved one predominates. "I am nothing without you"
- Decreases intelligence by distorting thoughts about love and the loved one. "Love makes you stupid"
- Euphoria, sleeplessness, lack of appetite, urgent energy and sexual desire overshadow everything else. "Love gives me wings"

Although it may not seem so, this phase is of great importance for the human species. Passion is an excellent evolutionary strategy that promotes multiple sexual encounters with the same person, thereby increasing the chances of having offspring and passing on our genes. Although falling in love consumes a lot of resources and limits one's ability to reason, it is the price we pay for survival of our species.

But in order to guarantee that same survival, infatuation must have a time limit, because if it were to last forever, the lovers, their offspring, and the species would be threatened. Who could raise a child in such a state? How could they identify a threat? For the sake of humanity, the passion of infatuation must subside, and give way to other stages of the couple's relationship or to new love stories.

Conscious love

After the temporary madness of falling in love, the biochemical framework changes. Our perception improves and we see the reality of love and the loved one, with all their lights and shadows. If we like what we see and the emotional bond that has been created is positive, levels of oxytocin, vasopressin and endorphins increase, generating feelings of calm, belonging and healthy attachment. Now we are talking about conscious love—the territory of intelligent, rational, and voluntary desire.

We have to understand that, contrary to how movies and novels portray love, conscious love is not created from romance, or from the discovery of a custom-made perfect partner. Conscious love arises from self-esteem and self-respect, and from this "self-love" a bond of personal and emotional growth is created with a partner we choose intelligently and rationally.

The desire created in conscious love can be as intense as active desire, but it stems from intelligence and calmness. Here, we are no longer overcome by hormones, but we control them. We build our love story and our desire day by day, by sharing pleasure, intimacy and emotions with commitment and dedication.

DESIRE IS FOR THOSE WHO WORK AT IT!

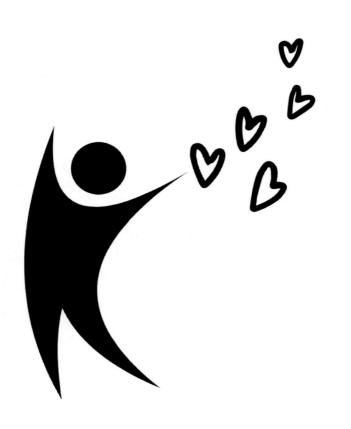

WHAT IS HAPPENING TO ME?

"What is not defined, cannot be measured. What is not measured, cannot be improved. What is not improved, is always degraded."

LORD WILLIAM THOMSON KELVIN

"Every morning I think: today will be different. But then — I don't know if it's laziness or just that I'm too tired, but I don't even let her touch me. I don't even look at her in case she gets turned on. At night she gets close to me and I pretend to be asleep so I don't have to reject her again. I love her with all my heart, but I don't feel like having sex. And I can't pretend, because she would know. It really upsets me, a lot. I'm afraid she'll end up leaving me because I don't give her what she needs."

Can you see yourself in this story? It is fictitious, but it is very similar to the stories we hear every day as sex therapists. Loss of sexual desire is one of the most frequent reasons for consulting a sexologist. 15% of all men and 30% of all women suffer from it. And this percentage is probably underestimated.

LOSS OF DESIRE IS A VERY COMMON PROBLEM!

Don't panic. It is normal for desire to fluctuate throughout our lives, especially throughout the course of a relationship. The fiery desire when we're falling in love eventually disappears. But it can be replaced by a reactive and conscious desire. And while this is a kind of desire that can be maintained and grow over time, it is also greatly impacted by life circumstances such as stress, illness, or emotional changes.

DESIRE CAN FLUCTUATE ENORMOUSLY OVER A LIFETIME.

It is only when this loss of desire persists over time and causes us discomfort that we face a problem to solve. And we must face it. Because loss of desire is a serious problem that can cause a lot of anguish, a lot of guilt, and a lot of fear, both for the person who suffers from it and for their partner, who feels rejected and unwanted.

For some time now, she rejects me every time I want to have sex. I understand that her work is very stressful, that she's tired, and that our day-to-day obligations are too much for the both of us, but she never touches me, kisses me, or even looks at me. I do my best to look nice, touch her, try to make her laugh and excite her, but nothing works. She doesn't even notice. I'm starting to give up on everything. I think it's my fault, that she just doesn't like me and isn't attracted to me anymore. Or maybe there's someone else. The truth is I'm very anxious because I know she'll end up leaving me.

I have heard testimonies like this one in different voices, genders, nationalities and ages, all full of anguish and asking for help. People who lose desire avoid intimacy and displays of affection so as not to reject their partner again. Even when sex happens and is enjoyed, the lack of interest in the sexual interaction is clearly perceived, and the rejected person may suffer as much, if not more, than the one who has lost desire. In fact, this continued sexual and affective rejection results in a loss of self-esteem that can be more painful than sexual dysfunction itself.

IN OTHER WORDS, IT IS NOT ONLY FREQUENT, BUT ALSO A SERIOUS PROBLEM!

¿Why does it happen?

Loss of desire can have many causes. It has what we call a multifactorial origin. Just one factor would be enough to cause it, but in most cases it's an accumulation of circumstances that come together to cause the problem.

Do you remember one of the opening scenes in The Mummy, where the main character is thrown off balance while placing a book in the Cairo museum library? The movement causes the bookshelf she has touched to fall, and with this, she causes the next one to fall and the next and the next, just like dominoes, until the whole Egyptian library is smashed in pieces to the ground. This is what happens to our desire when its pillars begin to fall, attacked by different factors.

You can watch the film's scene here:

https://youtu.be/rOZZeuGaQro

Stress

Stress is the most frequent cause of loss of desire. It can be caused by an excess of work commitments, family obligations, economic problems... When our minds are occupied with things that we consider more important than eroticism, we ignore the signals that turn us on. The pandemic we have suffered and the stress generated by medical and economic uncertainty have depleted many couples' libido.

Life changes

Age, motherhood and breastfeeding, caring for children or older relatives, menopause, bereavement. Life changes, however natural and physiological they may be, are not exempt from stress, anxiety, and problems that can lead to a loss of desire.

Toxic substances

Did you know that one of the main causes of sexual dysfunction is the abuse of toxic substances such as alcohol, tobacco, cannabis and other drugs? Please give them up. It will improve your desire, your orgasms, your sexuality and your health.

Boredom

It is logical for desire to decrease. What is boredom if not a lack of passion? We get bored if we always do the same thing, if we don't learn new erotic skills, if we don't look for other ways to enjoy and stimulate our eroticism.

Sexual and relationship problems

Lack of communication with the partner and the presence of sexual dysfunctions such as pain during intercourse or erectile dysfunction frequently cause loss of desire.

If you don't enjoy something, you don't want to repeat it. In addition, loss of desire worsens a couple's relationship and the intensity of sexual dysfunction, causing increasing discomfort.

Psychological problems

Many psychological problems can inhibit desire, but the most important are problems of self-esteem and body image, as well as a history of abuse and repressive upbringing. Unfortunately, these problems are so common that it is rare not to encounter them.

Medical problems and medication

All medical problems related to the physiology of sexual desire and response can cause its loss: hormonal, neurological and vascular disorders, as well as chronic diseases, such as cancer or psychiatric problems. We should also bear in mind that many treatments for these diseases reduce sexual desire.

Did you know that many of the most commonly prescribed drugs in adulthood have a negative influence on sexual desire? Antidepressants and blood pressure medications significantly affect the entire sexual response. Often, simply changing the dosage or the product resolves the problem, so if you feel that your loss of desire is related to a medication you are taking, consult your doctor to consider a change. But never stop taking medication without professional medical advice!

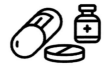

LET'S TAKE A TEST!

Don't worry, this is not a diagnostic procedure or a medical exam, it is just a 12-question test that will help you assess your current situation.

Take a pencil and answer "YES" or "NO" honestly and without thinking too much about it. Save the results; they're for you alone. It will help you identify how you are doing right now, and later, at the end of the book, to notice any changes that may have occurred.

If you answer "yes" to more than half of the questions, you have an issue with sexual desire. Write down your score. Let's see whether step by step, chapter by chapter, we can improve it.

1. Has your interest in sex decreased lately?

2. Have you stopped taking the initiative in sex?

3. Do you find excuses to avoid sex, or do you often refuse it?

4. Do you feel that the frequency of your sexual relations has decreased?

5. Do you feel that you are enjoying sex less?

6. Do you have problems with your partner because of the difference in your desire levels?

7. Have you stopped having sexual fantasies?

8. Do you masturbate less often than you used to, or not at all?

9. Do you think you could do without sex?

10. Do you avoid intimacy or talking about sex to avoid sexual interactions?

11. Do you feel less desirable than before?

12. Are you easily distracted during sex or look forward to it ending?

DO YOU REALLY WANT TO REAWAKEN YOUR DESIRE?

> *"When we are no longer able to change a situation, we are challenged to change ourselves."*
>
> VIKTOR FRANKL

Do you want to feel desire again? I would like you to think very carefully about your answer and if it is yes, I want you to say it out loud.

YES, I WANT TO FEEL DESIRE AGAIN

Repeat it louder, please.

YES, I WANT TO FEEL DESIRE AGAIN!

If your answer is affirmative, I assure you that you are reading the right book, because I have written it for you and for other people who want the same as you. However, if what you are looking for is to regain that irrational, hormonal desire we talked about in the first chapter, if you are interested in being eternally blinded by love, you better close this book and create an OK Cupid! account. As I have already explained, that kind of desire is not usually long-lasting (unless constantly finding new partners is your game plan) but that is not the subject of this book. Here we will talk about intelligent desire, which is built and worked on.

Do you remember my example about what causes the loss of desire? We compared it to the Egyptian museum shelves in The Mummy, that fell over one after the other, like dominoes. Well, just like in that museum, there is no magic wand that can lift the shelves all at once and put them back in order. The secret to getting them back into place is to lift them up one by one and reinforce them a bit, so that they're less likely to fall back down again. This is what I want you to do with your desire.

Where there is a will, there is a way

I was born in Santander. I studied medicine there and then I passed the MIR, the exam required for medical specialist training in Spain. I chose to train in Girona because it was one of the few places that had any vacancies left in Gynecology, which was what I wanted to study. Also because the sea was nearby (I can't live without having the ocean close to me) and because I had family in Barcelona whom I rarely saw. I was happy and excited to go there. But I hadn't realized that I would encounter a language barrier: I didn't speak a word of Catalan. And in Girona they speak it a lot. Although it was very difficult, I found wonderful friends who helped me and explained things to me. But I ran into someone who wasn't like most of them. It was shortly after I had arrived, on a day when I was in the operating room and I decided to speak in Catalan.

"Tisores, si us plau. (Scissors, please)"

The assistant smiled and handed them to me. She complimented me on my Catalan:

"Molt bé, Myriam. (Very good, Myriam)"

But the surgeon who was teaching me, and who didn't like me very much, said:

"No, no ho has dit bé i mai ho farás bé porque no ets d'aquí. Per parlar-lo així, millor que parlis en castellà. (No, you haven't said it well and you never will, because you're not from here. If you're going to speak like that, you'd better just speak in Spanish.)"

I reddened with anger under my mask but I didn't respond, and continued with the surgery. The next day I bought a pile of magazines, comics and books in Catalan to read. I stopped watching TV in Spanish and only watched TV3, the channel in Catalan. I started answering everyone in Catalan and asking them to please correct me. In less than six months I spoke it so well that the only question I sparked in the minds of those who spoke with me was which Catalan region my accent was from. And not only that. Today Catalan is my second language. I feel as Catalan as I do Menorcan and I love everything I have learned, shared and enjoyed there.

¿What am I trying to say with this?

First of all: that difficulties and rude people are excellent springboards for learning. As a popular saying goes:

EVERY KICK IN THE ASS IS A STEP FORWARD

The second thing is that motivation and hard work are the most important tools for getting what you want. If you want something, you can get it, but you have to work hard and eagerly. Remember: All you need is love. All you need is desire.

I don't plan to kick you in the ass, but I do want to motivate you and help you work on your desire.

ARE YOU WILLING TO DO YOUR PART?

ARE YOU WILLING TO WORK WITH LOVE?

SAY YES VERY LOUDLY!

The work plan

I am addicted to self-help and personal growth courses. I love them and I participate in a lot of them. However, a very curious thing used to happen to me in those workshops, and that is that I always learned much more slowly than the rest of the group – it would be very difficult for me and I often forgot almost everything I learned. However, this never happened to me in the medical courses I took on Gynecology, where I kept up the same pace as my classmates.

I couldn't understand this difficulty until I realized what was going on: I usually listened to the self-help courses when I had a bit of extra time or while I was doing something else. I never took notes and I didn't do the exercises and exams because they didn't count for my curriculum. Quite the opposite of what I did in my specialty: I had the Gynecology courses scheduled, I took notes all the time and then typed them up, I took all the exams, and if I could, I took them repeatedly in order to raise my grade.

Here was my explanation: although I loved the personal growth courses, I didn't give them the same importance I gave to the gynecology courses, nor did I work on them in the same way. That's why they took me much more effort and why I was less focused.

Now I set a schedule for all my courses, whatever they are. Each one has a notebook dedicated to it, where I write, draw, and design plans. I'm already so fast-paced that I even increase the speed of instructional videos to finish sooner and expand information in other ways. And the best part: what I learn, I never forget.

IF YOU WANT TO ACHIEVE SOMETHING, GIVE IT THE IMPORTANCE IT DESERVES AND SET YOURSELF A WORK PLAN TO IMPROVE YOUR DESIRE

The 7 steps

I'm sure you've heard that it takes four weeks to establish a habit. A well-known TV program in Spain argued that 21 days is enough. That is also what I've been told in many self-improvement courses. Why these figures? Apparently, before the moon landing in 1969, NASA conducted an experiment to measure the impact of weightlessness and the resulting space disorientation in astronauts. The study consisted of putting on convex glasses that inverted the image, turning it 180 degrees: it made them see the world upside down. They had to wear these glasses 24 hours a day, every day of the week. At first it created great anxiety and stress for them because of the lack of orientation that prevented them from doing their tasks properly. Some astronauts took off their glasses from time to time, but those who never took them off began to see everything un-inverted. The brain had completely adapted to this new world and had inverted the image. And this happened within four weeks of wearing them without a break. That is why four weeks became the magic number.

I've looked for this study and haven't found it. It doesn't appear in any medical library or on the NASA website. I have read several studies on the glasses experiment to demonstrate the great plasticity of our brain, but without any astronauts involved. I have also reviewed other studies that evaluate the time it takes to acquire habits, and I concluded that it is not an exact number, but that there is great variability for each person and for each activity, especially depending on how much we want to do it.

It is clear that there are no magic numbers, but all studies suggest that clarity of objectives, constancy and gradual learning facilitate the acquisition of habits.

This is why I have developed a 7-step plan in which week by week you will move toward your goal: reading, learning, writing and discovering how to improve your desire.

"It is necessary to vigorously shake the forest of dormant cerebral neurons; it is necessary to make them vibrate with the emotion of the new and to infuse them with noble and lofty concerns."

The notebook

Get yourself a notebook! Writing is the best way to clarify and consolidate ideas and knowledge, so get one. You can buy one you love, repurpose one you have, or even use a digital notebook. Write down everything that catches your attention, the ideas that you decide to put into action and all the reflections that the contents generate in you. Taking notes increases concentration and the ability to assimilate everything we learn, but also allows us to remember everything quickly after time has passed. So get a notebook NOW and put your name on it.

Commit!

If you've read this far, I have no doubt that you're interested in the subject. But being interested in a subject is not the same as being committed to it, just as being interested in a person is not the same as being committed to that person. If you want to receive what I offer you in this book, you have to dedicate your time and energy to it.

So I ask you the same question again:

ARE YOU REALLY WILLING TO WORK ON YOUR DESIRE?

Answer out loud.

YES, I AM WILLING TO WORK ON MY DESIRE

Louder!

YES, I AM WILLING TO WORK ON MY DESIRE!

Perfect! Because if you want to enjoy your desire again, if you want to grow sexually, you have to do your part. I don't have a magic wand to help you regain your desire, much less to fix a bad relationship. That wand is yours, and only yours, but you have to make it yourself. That is why I ask you to sign a symbolic document: a contract with yourself.

PERSONAL CONTRACT

I, [NAME] , hereby commit to:

- Reading "Rekindle Your Desire" in its entirety.
- Performing the exercises recommended in each step.
- Using what I learn to improve and explore my maximum erotic potential.
- Opening myself to new ways of changing and evolving.
- Not judging and not judging myself, respecting my own limits and those of others.
- Accepting that this path will require me to open my mind, to be brave and, maybe, to discover unexpected things.

SIGNATURE   DATE

STEP 1: KNOWLEDGE IS POWER

> *"Knowledge will make you be free."*
> SOCRATES

Learning allows us to grow, evolve and improve. Knowledge not only gives us more power, but also greater health and happiness. Education is so important that the UN considers it an essential human right, and protects it in its Universal Declaration of Human Rights.

EDUCATION IS VERY IMPORTANT AND IS A UNIVERSAL RIGHT

Do you agree with this? I'm sure you do. And I'm also sure that all the mothers throughout human history do as well, those who tell us:

"Study, read a lot and learn; that way you will become somebody."

"I'm going to sign you up for after-school classes so you'll do better than the others."

"The sooner you learn a bit about everything, the better"

You will have heard these phrases more than once. You may even have said them. However, look at what those same mothers say when the classes are about sexuality rather than French or math:

"Already? It's too soon, it's better if they explain this to you when you're older."

"Sex Education is good for nothing but to encourage you to have sex and touch yourself."

"All that stuff about sexual orientation does nothing but confuse you, and then unfortunate things start to happen."

Does this sound familiar to you? The fact is that they always want to play down the importance of Sex Education and contaminate it with fear. Fear! What we should be afraid of is sexual ignorance. You can't even imagine how much better the health of our girls and our society would be with a good Sex Education program from birth. Do you know that just by offering truthful and scientific sexual information, 80% of sexual problems could be solved? Learning about sexuality is so important that it is the first thing we are going to do. That's why our first step is called: KNOWLEDGE IS POWER.

"Education is the most powerful weapon which you can use to change the world"
NELSON MANDELA

Knowledge Is Power

Welcome to the first step of this book. In this chapter we are going to talk about some important concepts in sexuality. It's a bit more theoretical than the others, but don't be scared. I'm not going to give you a dense master class. I am convinced that you have already read everything and more on the subject.

But, I would like you to ask yourself one question: Are you convinced? Even if your intelligent brain is, we all have that irrational part that rebels against this kind of knowledge. It is that dark corner of the brain where monsters like myths and phobias grow, where you store what your grandmother told you when you were a child, what you heard on the street, or what you were told in the school bathroom. A theory might be very clear to you and you may understand the logic and science of it, but in practice, and especially when you go on autopilot, monsters appear. That is why it is important that we review a few things which I will point out, to see if this way, with a few big letters, we can chase those monsters away.

GOOD SEX IS GOOD FOR YOUR HEALTH

Yes! Absolutely! Yes, yes and yes. I will repeat this a million times: yes!!!

GOOD SEX IS GOOD FOR YOUR HEALTH

This has been scientifically proven. A healthy and positive sexuality makes us happier and more sociable, reduces stress, insomnia, chronic pain, and seems to impact the prevalence and better management of many conditions such as cardiovascular and oncological diseases. Sex, thanks to the release of some hormones such as DHEA (dehydroepiandrosterone), serotonin, endorphins and melatonin, improves the immune system, mood and physical health, is an analgesic and improves the pelvic floor. On the other hand, if the sexual experience is negative, it can cause health, psychological and relationship problems.

GOOD SEX IS GOOD FOR YOUR HEALTH

Sex is a source of well-being and pleasure. That is why I insist that good sex is good. And it is, even if there is no penetration, intercourse, or even orgasm, just pure satisfaction. Sexual health is so important to people's health that the World Health Organization (WHO) is firmly committed to guaranteeing it and to training health professionals to deal with it.

> "Sexual health is a state of physical, emotional, mental and social well-being in relation to sexuality. It requires a positive and respectful approach to sexuality and sexual relationships, as well as the possibility of having pleasurable and safe sexual experiences, free of coercion, discrimination and violence"

World Health Organization, 2002

The WHO affirms that achieving and maintaining the sexual health of the population requires respecting, protecting and guaranteeing the sexual rights of all people. And so it is.

But did you know that sexual rights were first enacted in Valencia in 1997? It is sad that this was so recent, when universal human rights were declared in 1948. Very sad. But society, religion and morality have created a lot of myths and lies about sexuality throughout history, probably for the sole purpose of social control. And don't think they've been eliminated. But I'm not going to talk to you about religions, morals or social norms. I leave those to you at home, just as I deal with mine. Here I will talk to you about science and common sense. And the fact is, to beat the dragon of myths, the only sword that works is that of science, reason and logic.

But to get to the point:

GOOD SEX IS GOOD FOR YOUR HEALTH

Of course, it's very good! How can good sex not be good if people with a vulva have an organ specialized only in pleasure? Evolution is austere and radical, eliminating everything that has no importance for survival. So, if there is a clitoris, whose only known function is pleasure, it is evident that pleasurable sex is important for our species, although this importance, like that of the clitoris, has been hidden from us for centuries.

So my friend, if good sex gives us health as well as power and happiness, it should be prescribed in every doctor's office. I, in fact, prescribe it.

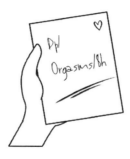

Everybody Has Sexuality

All human beings! And we have it throughout our lives. From the beginning to the end. From the moment we are born until we die. Because sexuality is an inseparable dimension of the human being that is present in everything we are, think, feel and do. Sexuality is not only eroticism and reproduction, it is also pleasure, gender, sex, orientation, identity, intimacy and love, expressed differently according to each person and in each moment of his or her life. Sexuality is always there, whether you have sex or not. You can't deny it, you can't remove it, you can't separate yourself from it. It influences your health and your mood. Because you are, like me and like everyone else, a sexual being.

Sex, Identity, Gender and Orientation

These are concepts that we often confuse and that confuse us. You can't even imagine how many times they are used in the wrong way, creating confusion and even discomfort. I will try to clarify them for you.

Sex

"Sex" is a generic term by which we usually refer to everything related to sexuality: having sex is sex, genitals are sex, our sexuality is what we think of as sex, and we categorize people according to sex, focusing only on male and female. But "sex" actually refers to the biological and genetic condition whereby we are born with male, female or combined sexual characteristics: that is, certain external sex organs, internal sex organs, chromosomes and hormones. That is sex.

SEX IS WHAT MY BODY IS LIKE

Society and science allowed itself to classify all people into one of two categories: male or female. In this way, people were "sexed" just like chicks, by placing them in one of two boxes: male or female. Most people, like the chicks, fit into one of those boxes without too much hesitation. And anything that could not be placed, because it did not fit into that classification, was considered abnormal.

Luckily today we know that what is abnormal is to pretend that all people are the same, given that all human beings are genetically and experientially different.

That science uses classifications is logical, since it is a way to record, learn and seek solutions to problems. It is the "scientific method". But we must NEVER forget that reality is much bigger and more diverse than a scientific study.

I'll explain it another way. Let's draw a line where we will put people with all-female biological, genetic, hormonal and physical characteristics at one extreme and all-male at the other.

Most people will put themselves somewhere between these two extreme biological definitions. A few, a very few, will be at the extremes: people who are physically very feminine or very masculine. Others will be in the middle: intersex people who share biological sex characteristics of both sexes. Intersexuality is not a disorder or a health problem, it is a natural human variation that, according to some studies, may be as frequent as 1 in 150 people.

My place on this line would be somewhere like this:

SEX

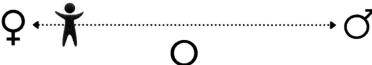

Biologically I am female and genetically too, but I am big and muscular and have a lot of hair, so I feel a bit removed from what would be the extreme biological female definition. That is why I place myself somewhat more to the right.

Where would you place yourself? Draw the sex line in your notebook and place yourself where you think you are situated. Write down why. Also write down your thoughts about what I have explained to you so far.

SEX

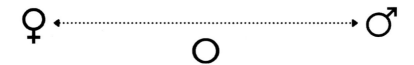

Gender or Gender Role

Just as sex is biological and physical, gender is expressive and behavioral. This behavior may be influenced by biology, but above all it is determined by your sociocultural environment and what society assigns and expects of you. Remember that these roles are "invented" by each society for each moment and each era. They are not standard.

GENDER IS HOW I BEHAVE

Just as in sex, each gender role—male and female—can be placed at either end of a line and all of us can place ourselves anywhere between the two extremes. Even if society doesn't expect me to be where I place myself, I assure you that any point is normal. And not only that, you can move from one point to another throughout your life, without that being abnormal or strange either.

Here I place where I feel my gender is.

GENDER

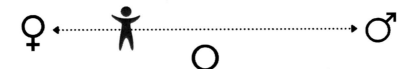

I have placed myself a little more to the right than in sex, and the fact is that, although my life's learning has made my gestures and behavior fulfill a feminine social role, there is a lot of masculinity in me: I am bossy, rebellious, independent; I do not like housework or fashion magazines; I wear little makeup... I love not meeting the standards of "my gender" because I do not agree with them at all.

Draw this line in your notebook and place yourself upon it. Write down which characteristics have made you place yourself there today. At another point in your life would you have placed yourself somewhere else?

GENDER

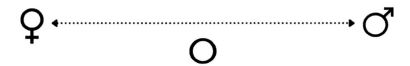

Gender Identity

This is the concept that is hardest for us to understand, because it is not visible like the previous ones. However, identity is truth, certainty, it is where and what you feel you are, both in terms of sex and gender.

IDENTITY IS WHAT I AM

In general, when one's feeling of identity coincides completely with their biological sex and gender, we call them a cisgender person. If it does not coincide at all, we speak of a trans person: transsexual if their identity does not coincide with their biological sex and transgender if it does not coincide with the gender role imposed by society. Many of us write trans*, instead of trans, to accommodate all possible options. Because it could also happen that a person does not identify with any gender or sometimes identifies more with one and then another. In this case we would be talking about non-binary or gender-fluid people.

Society usually applies the trans label to every person who has a conflict with his or her identity and uses various methods of transformation. However, trans people may not have any problem with their experience, and in fact, according to some theories, they would not have any problem at all if we were a healthy society that accepted all gender expressions.

Let's redraw a line for identity.

This would be mine:

IDENTITY

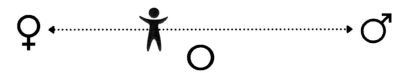

As you can see, although I do not consider myself absolutely feminine, my identity coincides with my sex and gender, so I define myself as cisgender.

Think about your own identity and place yourself where you stand on the line.

IDENTITY

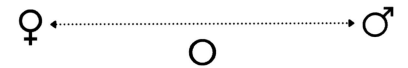

Write down your reflections.

Sexual Orientation

Now that you know how to differentiate sex, gender and identity, I want to tell you something that we often forget:

NEITHER YOUR SEX NOR YOUR GENDER DETERMINES YOUR ORIENTATION

Remember: whichever point on the sex or gender line a person occupies has nothing to do with their orientation. In other words, whether a person is more masculine or more feminine, either biologically (sex) or behaviorally (gender), has nothing to do with what they like.

ORIENTATION IS WHAT TURNS ME ON

Orientation is what each person likes: the affective and sexual attraction that people feel for each other. Since we love to classify things, we classify people according to their orientation, and we typically do so according to the distance between a person and the object of their desire on the masculine-feminine gender line. Let me explain: if my desire is usually directed toward people who are far away from me on the line, we call it heterosexuality. If, on the other hand, it is toward people who are very close to me, it is homosexuality. And if my desires are directed both near and far on the line, we speak of bisexuality.

ORIENTATION

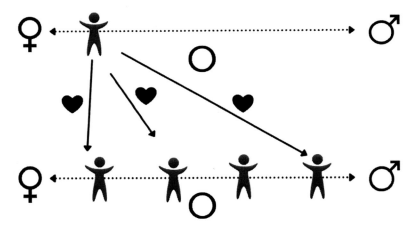

Of course, this is a very narrow classification. Reality is immensely diverse and we could define infinite orientations. For example:

⊖ Asexuality is characterized by the absence of interest in sexual relations with other people, although in some cases there may be romantic relations without eroticism.

⊖ Pansexuality is defined as attraction to other people regardless of their sex, identity or gender.

⊖ Demisexuality is an orientation in which there is only desire if there is an emotional bond.

⊖ Sapiosexuality is when desire is only stimulated by intellectual or moral qualities.

A person can identify with infinite orientations now and throughout his or her life, without that being a pathology, but something absolutely normal.

How do you define yourself right now? Write it down in your notebook and remember if and how it has changed throughout your life.

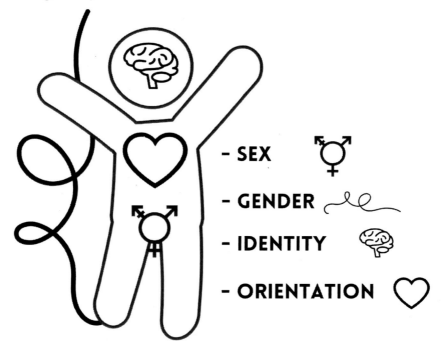

Sexual Response

The sexual response is a complex succession of physical, chemical and emotional changes that occur as a consequence of any form of sexual activity. These are not only genital changes, although those are the most striking, but changes in the whole body coordinated by hormones and neurotransmitters.

Each sexual response is unique and unrepeatable because it depends on our experience and thoughts, previous experiences, and the current moment. Therefore, we cannot speak of a single sexual response, but of infinite ways of responding.

THE SEXUAL RESPONSE IS UNIQUE AND VARIABLE IN EACH PERSON

But, although the sexual response is always different, in order to study it and above all to solve the problems that may appear, the wise men of Sexology have devised several models, of which you may have heard. All of them include differe... circular fashior

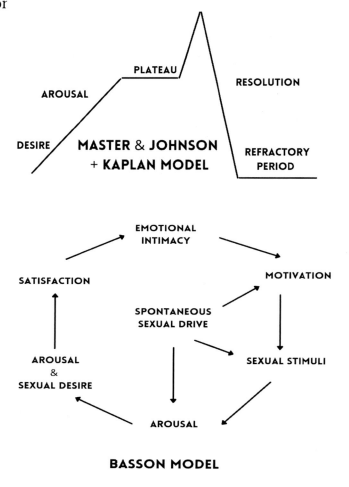

We could all fit into one of these, depending on where we're at in life. And we may even have a unique and particular response cycle that doesn't fit into any of them. That's normal! But it is very useful for you to know the most important phases, even if you don't experience them all or not in the order in which they are appear in the classic models.

The best known phases are desire, arousal and orgasm. The most important is satisfaction.

Desire

What am I going to tell you about desire? We have dedicated this book to it and we have discussed it extensively in these first chapters. We can have spontaneous desire, reactive to stimuli, or to sexual arousal itself, which in itself is capable of increasing desire.

Arousal

In this phase there is an increase in blood flow to the genitals, generally in response to stimuli. This increased blood flow to the area produces, among other things, changes in the color, shape and size of the genitals, vaginal lubrication and erection of the clitoris and penis. It also increases the heart and respiratory rate.

Orgasm

Orgasm is a set of physical and emotional sensations that occur after the discharge of accumulated sexual tension and cause a transitory sensation of pleasure, well-being and satisfaction.

During orgasm many physiological changes occur: vaginal, uterine, anal and penile contractions, muscle spasms, genital vasocongestion. Ejaculation can occur during orgasm, whether you have a penis or a vulva.

There are no different orgasms because you have a penis or a clitoris, nor because what is stimulated is the glans, the vagina or the anus. Orgasms are always different because they are a cerebral response of intense pleasure to an arousal that can always be different and come from anywhere: the clitoris, the penis, the vagina, the nipples, the mouth, the imagination, erotic dreams? Have you never woken up in the middle of an orgasm?

Sexual Satisfaction

I have told you that this is the most important phase and that's because it is the one that best relates to your physical, psychological, and couple's health. Sexual satisfaction is the result of evaluating the positive and negative aspects of the sexual interaction you have had.

This is the final grade you ascribe to how you felt. But not because of the intensity of an orgasm or the most gymnastic position. Satisfaction can be a 10 without having had an orgasm, or without having even moved. It is very subjective and variable, and above all reflects having achieved what we want. Satisfaction is reflected more in the final sigh than in the intensity of the orgasm.

Masturbation Is Normal and Healthy

Masturbating (touching yourself for sexual pleasure) is totally normal, whether you have sex with other people or not. Everyone masturbates differently and for different reasons. There are those who masturbate frequently, those who masturbate once in a while, and even those who never masturbate at all. All of this is fine, as long as it's what someone feels like doing, and is not forced by anyone or anything.

Although masturbation has been punished and censored throughout history through myths and erroneous beliefs, science has shown that masturbation is not bad, but the opposite: IT IS VERY GOOD. And the fact is that masturbating liberates, improves mood, is anxiolytic, analgesic, pleasurable and essential for sexual learning, which never ends.

Masturbation improves concentration and intellectual and creative capacity, increases sexual desire and vitality, tones the pelvic floor, improves genital dryness and strengthens the immune system. Masturbation improves the intensity of orgasms in couples, promotes self-knowledge, reduces stress, decreases insomnia and promotes emotional and mental stability.

MASTURBATION IS NORMAL, SAFE AND HEALTHY

Copy this sentence in capital letters three times in your notebook, please.

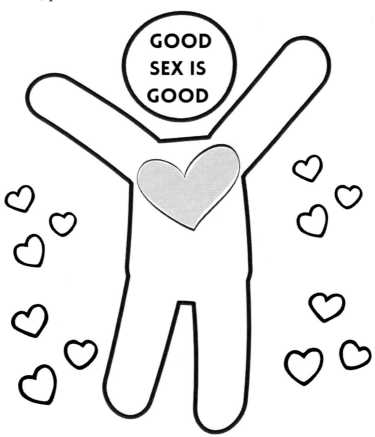

STEP 2: I LOVE ME

"If you don't love yourself, you might accept a type of love that is less than what you deserve."

FRIDA KAHLO

Welcome to the second step. I'm so glad you're still here, because you're going to love this step and you're going to learn a lot of things about yourself. First of all, I would like you to answer these questions:

- Do you like to look in the mirror several times a day?
- Are you comfortable sharing your opinion when it is different from others'?
- Do you get angry if you are not told that you've done things right?
- Do you beat yourself up when you make a mistake?
- Are you easily upset by criticism?
- Do you get stuck in a loop, thinking about it a thousand times, when something doesn't go the way you expected? Do you think you are always unlucky?
- If you indulge yourself, do you do it on the sly?
- Are you jealous?

⊖ Are you overwhelmed by being alone? When you are alone, do you work or watch TV non-stop?

If you have answered yes to more than five questions, I'm afraid you urgently need to start loving yourself, because right now you don't.

Think about this and tell me: why don't you love yourself? Who told you that you are not worthy of love? Do you believe that first you have to love others, and then, if it comes to it, yourself?

My psychologist friend, Gaby Paoli, a great therapist and a better co-teacher, always makes us laugh in her workshops, when she pretends to speak to us like a flight-attendant:

" Put on your oxygen mask before helping others."

In the event of cabin depressurization, we only have 15 seconds to start breathing before falling unconscious. And if you don't put it on your mask and breathe, if you're not at 100%, you're not helping yourself or anyone else.

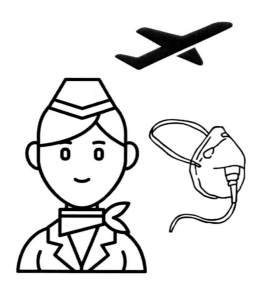
o

Apply this principle to real life: Don't you want to give the best of yourself? Don't you want the best of everything for the people you love? Well, the better you are, the greater you will be able to give, because you can't give what you don't have.

As a great Christian saying goes:

LOVE THY NEIGHBOR AS THYSELF

And if you do not love yourself enough, if you do not pamper and care for yourself, you will not be able to give much to others.

TO LOVE THY NEIGHBOR THOU MUST LOVE THYSELF

Rosa's Wedding is a movie from 2020 that I loved. If you haven't seen it, try to find it. It's directed by Icíar Bollaín and Alicia Luna, and the main character is played by my beloved Candela Peña: I've been a total fan since I met her ages ago in Barcelona, before I came to Menorca. Candela plays the role of Rosa, an endearing woman who lives, like many women, for her family, friends, neighbors, work... Then one day she decides to get married. To herself!

Have you ever heard of this? It's called sologamy and it's nothing new. It's a practice that has more and more followers and there are already companies that take care of organizing everything for you to enjoy a solo wedding in style.

It is wonderful to see how Rosa gets married. Her wedding vows moved me. The bride said something like this:

- Today I have decided to commit to myself, because to be treated with respect and love, you have to respect and love yourself.

- I promise to respect and care for myself.

- I promise to listen and forgive myself.

- I promise to do what is good for me, and not just for others.

- I promise to carry out my dreams and desires.

- I promise to love myself with all my heart all the days of my life.

- I renounce putting my happiness in the hands of others.

⊖ And I renounce being obedient.

Repeat these vows slowly and out loud, please. Reflect on them. What do you feel? I cried when I did it. Did the same happen to you?

Why is it so hard for us to make these promises to ourselves? Why is it almost impossible to live up to them?

I would like more and more people to decide to marry themselves, even if in less elaborate ceremonies than Rosa's.

To love oneself, as well as to love another person, it is not enough to just say it. Love is felt, shown and demonstrated. And how is this accomplished? Well, with small gestures of appreciation, respect and care. And that is what you have to give yourself. That's what you have to do: take care of yourself, pamper yourself, and love yourself.

TREAT YOURSELF THE WAY YOU WOULD TREAT YOUR BEST FRIEND

LOVE YOURSELF THE WAY YOU LOVE YOUR BEST FRIEND

In this step we are going to talk about a few essential things for taking care of ourselves and loving ourselves more. But first, I want you to write in your notebook, very visible, in big, beautiful letters:

I LOVE ME

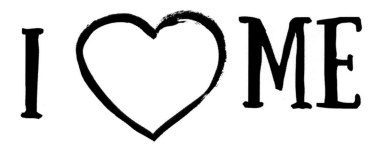

At the Top of Your Lungs

The coronavirus pandemic has taught us many things, and one of them is the importance of the oxygen level in the environment. Purifying devices and air quality meters have proliferated. The fact is that if we are well oxygenated, we are more active, and all our bodily systems work better. That is why it is essential to breathe clean air with adequate levels of oxygen. So, always ventilate your home well, as recommended during the lock-down (you can learn from everything), and avoid polluted environments, smoke and tobacco as much as possible.

VENTILATE YOUR HOUSE AND AVOID FUMES

Not only does it matter what you breathe, how you breathe also matters a lot. When I told this to a friend she replied:

"Come on, Myriam. I've been breathing for fifty years and I'm still alive, I can't be that bad at it."

And she was partially right. She breathed well enough to survive. But what if I told you that you could breathe to live better? Or even heal? Wouldn't you like to change that?

Although we breathe unconsciously, we don't always breathe the same way. Notice how you breathe when you are relaxed in bed. Try it now. If you can, lie down for a moment, close your eyes and observe your breathing for a few minutes. Compare it to the way you breathe when you are standing, walking, talking or working. Take a walk and observe again how you breathe. It's nothing like your breathing while lying down, is it? And it's not like your breathing in a state of relaxation. In times of activity or stress, breathing is shallow and fast, while when you are relaxed you breathe slowly, intensely and deeply.

This is very interesting because it also works the other way around. If you do this type of breathing on purpose, besides oxygenating more, you will induce your mind to relax. Slow, deep breathing is one of the best ways to reduce stress, because it sends an immediate message of calm to the brain, which in turn sends that message to the whole body. By receiving this message of calm, all the bodily changes that may have been set in motion by stress, such as tachycardia, sweating, or hypertension, are normalized, further increasing a feeling of calmness.

BREATHING INFLUENCES YOUR BODY AND YOUR STATE OF HEALTH.

Breathing Exercises

Breathing exercises are an excellent, easy and practical way to relax, reduce tension and relieve stress. They are easy to learn and you can do them whenever you want. You will find many deep breathing exercises online, many of them connected with meditation and yoga techniques. All of them are wonderful, so I encourage you to explore them. Here are a few simple exercises to establish as initial rituals of self-love.

1- Deep Breathing

Put one hand on your chest and one on your abdomen. Inhale slowly up to your maximum, taking the air slowly without raising your shoulders, bringing it towards your pelvis and feeling your belly swell. Slowly release all the air and notice how the abdominal hand descends.

Repeat 3 times.

2- Breathing in Phases 4-4-4

This consists of breathing in three distinct phases: inhalation, air retention, and exhalation. It allows greater control over and depth of your breathing. Inhale slowly, counting mentally 4 seconds. In the beginning, you can calculate the time with the stopwatch of your cell phone, then you will progressively learn the rhythm. Hold your breath for another 4 seconds and exhale for another 4 seconds.

- Inhale 1...2...3...4
- Retain 1...2...3...4
- Exhale 1...2...3...4

Repeat 3 times.

3- Breath Counting

In addition to relaxing, this exercise helps you gain awareness. It consists of breathing slowly and deeply, taking as many breaths as you can before you become distracted. At the beginning, you will lose the number very soon, but each time you practice, you will increase the amount. Set a goal for yourself to breathe 100 times without getting distracted.

1-2-3-4-5-6-7-8-9-10-11-12-13-14-15-16-17...

If you have not done these three breathing exercises while reading the instructions, practice them now. Write any changes you notice after doing them in your notebook.

I recommend that you always do one breathing exercise in the morning, another one at night, and whenever you feel anxious. You will see that they're such a simple way to lower your anxiety levels.

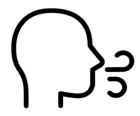

Hydrate!

I'm sure that at some point you've gone blank and said "I have it on the tip of my tongue! Do you know that maybe this wasn't because of a lapse of memory, but because of a lack of water? Dehydration decreases intellectual performance, attention and concentration, and it does so before you know you're thirsty! But it also causes fatigue, headaches, constipation, dry skin, and joint pain. You can even die from dehydration.

Water is necessary for most of our bodily functions. It helps us regulate temperature, eliminate toxins and transport substances. It boosts the immune system, increases metabolism and slows skin's aging.

Water accounts for 60% of our weight and we have no capacity to store it, so it all depends on what you drink. Every day you lose about two and a half liters through breathing, sweating, urine and feces, so this should be the minimum amount you should take in every day. 80% comes from drinking water and only 20% through food, so the recommendation is to drink at least two liters daily. A rule of thumb is to drink 8 glasses of water a day; more if you are older, hot, sick, or do a lot of exercise. Water intake should happen gradually throughout the day.

Record the amount of water you drink during a normal day in your notebook. Try to drink the recommended amount for a week and observe any changes in your activity, skin, and concentration. You may discover other positive effects of being better hydrated. Write them down and underline them, so you don't forget their importance.

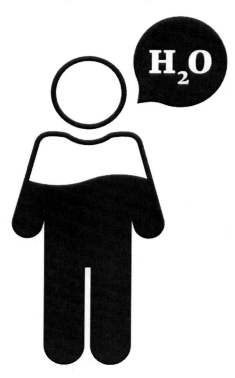

Eat Right

As we mentioned in the first step, the sexual response is influenced by multiple biological, physical and psychological factors. So it is logical to think that, if we have a healthy diet and appropriate intake of nutrients, the functions of all bodily systems will benefit. And so it is. Healthy nutrition habits are related to a better state of health, energy, and vitality, positively impacting the libido and sexual appetite.

And what is healthy eating? Well, it is a balanced, varied and appropriate diet for you: tailored to your needs and preferences, with all the essential nutrients, without deficits or excesses, and avoiding processed foods. Industrial or processed foods can cause health problems that influence sexuality, such as obesity, hypertension and diabetes, but also often contain substances that mimic or become hormones and interfere with sexual response.

What if I take aphrodisiacs?

Surely you have heard of foods that increase sexual appetite: oysters, honey, ginger, avocado, banana, walnuts, caviar, strawberries…

Unfortunately, there is no scientific evidence that they produce this effect, although just because they have this reputation, are energizing, and activate our senses through visual or gastronomic pleasure, they are indeed a good idea for a romantic dinner or as a prelude to a sexual interaction.

What you might not know is that there are also foods that are linked to a loss of desire: the so-called anaphrodisiacs or anti-aphrodisiacs. There is no hard scientific evidence for this either, but it is quite logical, because many of them are sedatives or cause bad breath or gas: hops, alcohol, tobacco, onions… Some of them can have the same deterrent effect as flip-flops with socks.

Are you eating a healthy diet? Don't hesitate to consult a nutrition professional to help you answer this question and give you advice.

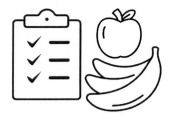

Get Moving

Physical exercise improves our health, makes us feel better, and also increases our libido. Physical activity enhances well-being for various reasons: it releases endorphins (chemical substances that produce pleasure), improves mood, strengthens vitality, and increases satisfaction with one's own body. But it also improves vigor and sexual capacity: you perform better and you enjoy more. And when you enjoy more, you want more.

It's not just a matter of logic: there is scientific evidence that erotic desire is positively linked to physical exercise.

PHYSICAL EXERCISE INCREASES DESIRE

Although everyone knows that exercise is good for your health, there are still too many people who don't do enough of it. According to the US Centers for Disease Control and Prevention, more than 60% of adults do not engage in the recommended amount of physical activity.

Did you know that just 30 minutes of moderate exercise five days a week significantly reduces the risk of diabetes, cancer and cardiovascular problems? Just a simple half-hour walk is enough! Plus, you'll reduce stress, have more energy and guess what: your desire will improve.

What are you waiting for to start?

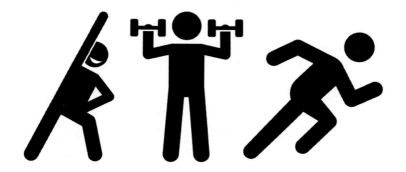

Train Your Pelvic Floor

There's a lot of talk about the health benefits of pelvic floor exercises for everyone, but did you know that they can also improve desire?

In 1940, gynecologist Arnold Kegel developed a plan of voluntary pelvic floor contraction exercises to treat urinary incontinence in his patients after childbirth. Kegel's exercises were shown to improve incontinence, but they also had an added benefit: they increased orgasms!

In fact, it was only logical, since sexual response is influenced by the same anatomical and vascular factors that were improved by the exercises.

Whether it's the simple—but effective—Kegels, such as vaginal spheres, biofeedback exercises and hypopressive abdominals, or a custom training program devised by a professional, what is clear is that taking care of and exercising the pelvic floor will improve your entire sexual response and therefore your desire.

Stronger and healthier pelvic floor muscles will improve your genital sensitivity and the intensity of arousal and orgasm independent of your genitalia.

PROPER PELVIC FLOOR EXERCISE IMPROVES SEXUAL RESPONSIVENESS

I will describe the Kegel exercises. But remember, if you have a pelvic floor problem, do not hesitate to contact a good physiotherapist.

How to do KEGEL exercises

⊖ First locate your pelvic floor. You can do this by interrupting the urinary flow when you go to pee. Do not do it out of habit, you should only do it to learn to identify it and not as a regular exercise.

⊖ If you have a vagina, you can finish locating your pelvic floor by inserting a lubricated finger into the vagina, to feel the contraction of its walls when you contract the pelvic area.

⊖ If you have a penis, touch your perineum and notice how it contracts and how the testicles rise when you contract it.

⊖ Once you have identified your pelvic floor muscles, get into a position where it is easy to identify or touch them as you contract them. To begin with, it is usually easiest lying on your back. Whichever position you choose, always remember to keep your back straight and relaxed, breathe calmly and do not contract any other muscles, neither buttocks nor abdomen muscles.

⊖ Contract and lift the pelvic floor muscles as if you were picking up and lifting the pelvic organs towards your navel. Hold the contraction for a few seconds. Relax slowly and contract again.

⊖ Do three sets of 8 contractions.

Doing the Kegels will only take a few minutes a day. Make it routine. You can increase the intensity and speed as you train and do more complex exercises each time.

Many studies in physical therapy, gynecology and sexology have shown that training the pelvic floor muscles improves genital sensitivity and hydration, erection, vascularization, intensity of arousal and orgasms. And if the result is more satisfying, desire improves!

Think about your pelvic floor. Plan how you want to improve it and what you will do to achieve this. Choose the time of day that you will dedicate to your pelvic floor. You can do it during a routine activity like watching TV or riding the bus, but it's also great to entirely dedicate a moment to your own pleasure and orgasms.

As I said, a healthy pelvic floor improves orgasms, but an orgasm exercises the pelvic floor in the most pleasurable way possible.

A TRAINED PELVIC FLOOR IMPROVES ORGASMS

ORGASMS IMPROVE THE PELVIC FLOOR

Get Organized

Organization is essential! An organized mind promotes a healthy life and reduces stress, the Number One Enemy of desire.

It's not about tidying up your house as if you were Marie Kondo or downloading the latest mobile app to organize your to-do lists. There are many very useful and widely recommended techniques, and I use many of them, but to begin, you just need to sit down and think calmly about what you can do to better organize yourself. Because getting organized is very important.

GETTING ORGANIZED IS ESSENTIAL

Did you know that having endless to-do lists and daily activities can kill you? Yes, you read that right: kill you! The stress that it generates and all its negative neurohormonal effects lead to bad habits, obesity, cardiovascular diseases and of course: sexual problems.

ADVANTAGES OF BEING ORGANIZED

- ϴ You will have more free time.
- ϴ You will develop greater concentration.
- ϴ You will increase your creativity.
- ϴ You will maintain more healthy habits.
- ϴ You will not forget anything.

- You will not lose anything.
- You will have less stress.
- You will be more productive.
- You will have more confidence.
- Your energy will increase.
- Your desire will improve.

How to get organized?

There are entire libraries about how to get organized. Multitasking, stress, and lack of time are part of our daily lives. You can find a lot of interesting methods and organizational gurus on the internet. Take a look and assess whether any method works with your reality. No one really knows what you need better than you do.

But, for starters:

- Free up your brain. Get a planner. Digital, or on paper, even if it's just four stapled pages. Your phone's Notes app will also suffice. Choose what you want, but write down your pending tasks and free up your memory. The brain is made to be creative, not to make lists or remember appointments.

- Organize your tasks: by priority, by time, by topic. Assign each a day and time, being very realistic.

- Do one task at a time. The brain is not designed to focus on more than one thing at a time, and when it has to do so, it is not only less efficient, but also generates a lot of stress. When you are engaged in something, do only that and avoid distractions. Especially when you engage in sex. Please.

- Tidy up and simplify: your house, your cellphone, your computer, your life... Get rid of anything you don't need or does not make you happy.

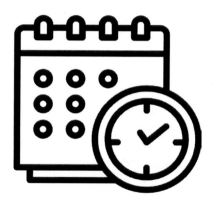

Sleep Well

Poor sleep is so common that it seems normal to us. Many people who do not sleep because of their work often say: "I'll sleep when I'm dead." What they don't know is that, if they don't sleep, eternal rest may come sooner than they think.

Lack of sleep is related to diseases that can reduce your quality of life and life expectancy, such as obesity, hypertension, anxiety, depression, heart attack and dementia.

As if this were not enough, poor sleep also leads to sexual dysfunction, decreasing arousal, erections, the intensity of orgasms, and of course: desire.

How to improve your rest?

ϴ Go to sleep at the same time every day.

ϴ Avoid stimulants such as tea and caffeine at night.

ϴ Eat a light dinner.

ϴ Get 30 minutes of moderate exercise each day.

ϴ Disconnect from screens at least half an hour before bedtime.

ϴ Turn off your cell phone, or store it away from the bed. Its light alters the quality of your sleep.

ϴ Do not smoke, or at least avoid smoking before going to sleep.

ϴ Choose a comfortable and quiet place to rest.

⊖ Remember what is most conducive to restful sleep: an orgasm!

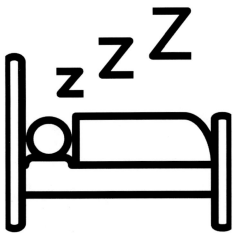

Drop the Toxins

Did you know that eliminating toxins from your life will improve your sex? I am not referring to toxic people, who also deserve it, but to alcohol, tobacco, cannabis and other drugs.

Simply reducing them will increase your sexual capacity, improving all phases of your response and therefore also your desire.

Have Fun!

The word "leisure" comes from the Latin "otium" which means rest. We know that rest is necessary for your health, and this not only refers to sleep, but also to leisure. Healthy leisure helps you maintain good health, reduces stress, improves energy levels and also efficiency. In fact, there are already many companies, such as Google, that encourage their employees to enjoy breaks and downtime with meditation or games to improve their work performance.

Leisure is good for your health, and therefore, for your desire, but beware, it also has a dark side, since on the one hand we can mix fun with toxins and risky behaviors, or we can become saturated and stressed by an excess of extracurricular activities: concerts, outings, ceramics courses, yoga workshops... Don't let your leisure time stress you out either! Look for a healthy activity that makes you happy, smile, and above all, laugh.

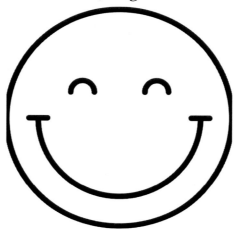

I'll go over it all again so you don't forget:
- BREATHE GOOD AIR AND DO BREATHING EXERCISES
- HYDRATE
- EAT WELL
- EXERCISE AND BREATHE
- TRAIN YOUR PELVIC FLOOR WELL
- GET ORGANIZED
- GET GOOD SLEEP
- STOP USING TOXIC SUBSTANCES
- ENJOY YOUR FREE TIME

Write again in your notebook:

I LOVE ME

And add:

I TAKE CARE OF MYSELF

I hope you have written it with conviction. Because I hope I have convinced you of how important it is to love and care for yourself. For you, for your health, for your desire, and for the health and desire of all the people you love.

Make a list of all the new things this chapter has inspired you to start doing, either because you need them or because you find them interesting. Set a date to start doing them.

And to finish this second step I would like you to do one last thing... can you guess it??

MARRY YOURSELF!

You don't need to have a reception, although it would be a great idea to get together with some friends. But what I do ask is that you write your own wedding vows. You can be inspired by Rosa's.

Write them or print them beautifully, place them in a visible spot and read them out loud every day.

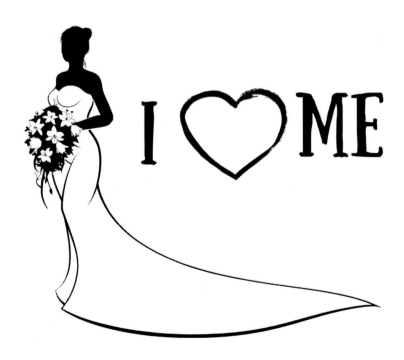

STEP 3: YOU SEXY THING

"I believe in miracles
Where're you from?
You sexy thing (sexy thing you)
I believe in miracles
Since you came along
You sexy thing"

Hot Chocolate: You Sexy Thing

Sexy

According to the dictionary, "sexy" refers to someone who exerts or possesses physical and sexual attractiveness, or to physical and sexual attractiveness itself. In general, we usually associate "sexy" with physically attractive people, but we all know people with divine features and bodies who don't do it for us, while others, who might not meet any of the damn aesthetic ideals, attract all the looks and sighs.

That is because being sexy is more an attitude than a physical trait, and do you know what the advantage of attitude over physical trait is? It can be learned.

Welcome to the third step of the book, in which we are going to fill your life with "sexy" through several powerful strategies.

Are you ready?

Think Sexy

People say I am very cheerful and optimistic, but how could I not be? Life has rewarded me by putting wonderful people by my side, the kind that improve you and make you grow. One of them is my captain, my boss and my teacher Josep Fulquet. Although we worked together more than two decades ago, I remember every conversation with him as if it were yesterday.

One day we got to talking about one of the most frequently asked questions in an OB-GYN's office. Can you guess what it's about? Yes, desire. At the time I was an absolutely analytic doctor who searched for all the answers and remedies for my patients in the pharmacopoeia, traditional or alternative. But he, prudent and perceptive as always, said to me:

"Maybe some of those things you look for in the handbook will help, but Myriam, to not lose desire what you have to do is not to let go of it. You have to think more about sex, because sex evokes sex. If you don't want to lose desire, you have to always keep it on your mind."

And that's the way it is. My boss was absolutely right. We put sex in a corner because of day-to-day obligations and we do this so much that it ends up disappearing from our minds. That's why the first exercise I'm going to recommend you to do in this chapter is: think sexy.

But how can we think more about sex?

To start, find a comfortable, quiet place and open your precious desire notebook. Close your eyes, take a couple of deep breaths, and go back in your memory....

Let's start at the beginning. What is your first memory of sexual arousal? What triggered it? Did it feel good? If the memory is positive, write it down and describe it in as much detail as possible.

If you have remembered others and they are nice, write them down too. Write down all the good things you remember.

Take another deep breath and close your eyes. Now rewind to the most satisfying sexual interaction you remember, whether alone or in company, and whoever the company was. Write it down and describe it in detail as well.

If you can't decide which one is the most satisfying, write down all the ones that might be candidates for it. Do not spare anything in the descriptions.

Reread everything you've recorded. How do you feel about it? Write that down too, and think about what you could improve and what you would have liked to add.

Everything you've written down is now part of your erotic memory. Keeping the positive part of that memory in mind will help you to activate your libido and, above all, will give you a very useful tool to be able to work on your desire.

Don't stop here! Research, remember, look at pictures, ask questions... Collect all your positive erotic memory. Put it in your notebook, but consider whether you could dedicate a whole notebook to it in the future. Or if you could even set up a "sexy bookshelf" at home.

Enrich Your Sexy

Eroticism is the form of expression of sexuality that is directed toward the pursuit of intimacy and sexual pleasure. It encompasses fantasies and desires as well as sexual interactions and relationships.

The need for erotic expression is universal, but it varies according to culture, each of which sets different limits and rules. There are cultures that are very restrictive with people who have a vulva, not allowing them any erotic expression. And there are those, like ours, that are reluctant to acknowledge the erotic expression of non-normative people, that is, those people who are outside the established norms of age, gender, beauty and orientation.

In addition to sociocultural influence, each person sets his or her own particular rules regarding eroticism, being more restrictive or permissive depending on his or her way of thinking and learning. There are people who may find it very embarrassing to show their arousal or talk openly about sex, and others who are most aroused by showing it and by explicit and foul language. There are those who never reveal themselves, while others heat up the atmosphere just by blinking.

Everything is valid, as long as it is what feels good to you and what you choose. Remember that erotic expression is learned and chosen, so it can evolve and you can change it every day of your life.

If you enrich it, the evolution will always be for the better.

But how can eroticism be enriched?

Well, one way is to record your erotic memory, as we have learned to document in the previous section. But the fastest and most effective way to enrich it are fantasies, yours and those of others, and expressed in all possible ways, from oral language to the most sublime artistic manifestations.

Now let's talk about fantasies, erotic literature, erotic cinema and audio porn.

FANTASIES

Let's start with your own fantasies. Take out your notebook and close your eyes. Think of the first sexual fantasy that comes to mind. Do you like it? Then give it a title and write it down. Describe it in detail: what it is, why, how it is, where it happens, in what situation, how you enjoy it... If you feel like it, decorate the story with a drawing or an illustrative photo.

Can you think of any other fantasy? If so, describe it too, but if not, that's ok too. You will come up with many more as you read the book, fantasies are like eating peanuts -- once you start you can't finish. When they appear, write them down. Didn't I tell you you'd end up with a sexy library?

EROTIC LITERATURE

Literature is a fantastic resource for erotic fantasies. There is nothing that sparks the imagination and enriches our fantasies more than stories.

Open your notebook. Let's make a list of erotic literary resources. I'm sure you remember books that have stimulated your eroticism. Write them all down.

I'm going to give you examples of some classics and some more modern ones in case they inspire you.

- Delta of Venus, by Anaïs Nin.
- Story of the eye, by George Bataille.
- The Lover, by Marguerite Duras.
- Story of O, by Pauline Reage.
- Emmanuelle, by Emmanuelle Arsan.
- Ada, or Ardor: A Family Chronicle, by Vladimir Nabokov.
- Lady Chatterley's Lover, by D.H. Lawrence.
- The Ages of Lulu, by Almudena Grandes.
- In Valeria's shoes, by Elisabet Benavent.
- Unwrap Me: A Stark Ever After Novella, by Julie Kenner.
- Outlander, by Diana Gabaldon.
- Ask Me What You Want, by Megan Maxwell.
- Masters and Dungeons, by Lena Valenti.
- Fifty Shades of Grey, by E.L. James.
- Bared to You, by Sylvia Day.
- Night Shift, by Joanna Angel.
- Evil Angels, by Pascal Bruckner

You can find many pages dedicated to erotic fiction on the internet, where new authors publish their stories. If you feel like it, google "erotic literature" and enjoy. You will find all kinds of themes.

SEXY MOVIES

Now we come to cinematic art. Try to remember movies that have turned you on or inspired erotic fantasies.

Don't be surprised if some adventure movies or romance stories may have turned you on. They might have wonderful scenes to inspire your fantasy diary. Think, for example, of:

- Love Story.
- Call Me By Your Name.
- Blue Lagoon.
- The Notebook.
- Ghost.
- Brokeback Mountain.
- From Here to Eternity.

Other films contain very explicit sex scenes although they are not classified as porn:

- Bound.
- Blue Is the Warmest Color.
- Eyes Wide Shut.
- Y Tu Mamá También.
- Sex and Lucía.
- Nine Songs.

And of course, I should at least mention the all-time star of visual fantasy: porn. By pornography or porn we refer to material that represents sexual or erotic acts with the purpose of provoking sexual arousal in the spectator. Porn movies are made for that purpose.

And yes, watching porn is a good way to increase your arousal and desire, even though it may seem negative at first.

Why do we think porn is bad? Well, because it often is, and can be for many reasons:

- Because it denigrates, exploits and mistreats the actors, and especially the actresses.
- Because it can show negative, sexist, violent, misogynist and homophobic sexual behaviors.

⊖ Because it only teaches normative bodies and behaviors, far from reality.

⊖ Because it is considered a platform for sexual learning, instead of a fiction, which is what it is. As Lyona says in her book Sex Oh!, learning sex from porn is like learning to drive by watching Fast & Furious.

⊖ Because its cinematic quality is often very bad.

Fortunately, there is more interest nowadays in making more ethical and higher quality porn, which addresses diverse realities, ages, genders and bodies. A more interesting and healthy porn, even if it remains what it is: fiction to eroticize.

I'm sure you'll find porn movies that you'll like to watch on the internet and pay-per-view platforms. The works of directors like Erika Lust, Irina Vega or Shine Louise Houston are quite interesting.

If you feel like it, do your research on such wonderful platforms as: Lust Cinema, Else Cinema, The Alternative Porn Community, Ersties, Four Chambers, or Pink Label.

Write all the movie titles and platforms that interest you in your notebook. Research them. Highlight the scenes that have most aroused your libido and describe them. Keep expanding your "sexy shelf."

AUDIO PORN

Everything is more erotic when whispered in the ear. It is only logical that, with the rise of podcasts and audiobooks, eroticism would also be looking for its sonorous version. And not only has it discovered it, audio porn has taken off and become one of the most downloaded types of content during the 2020 pandemic confinement. Audio porn, or porncasts, merge erotic literature and podcasts and provide new tools for arousing us and stimulating our desire.

I recommend that you visit Dipsea at dipseastories.com, Quinn at tryquinn.com or Fearly at weare-ferly.com. These platforms were the first to break into audioeroticism and stand out for their diverse, healthy and gender-sensitive content.

Have you made good note of everything? Yes? Because you have just expanded what we call the sexual-erotic imaginary. Your own. And not only that, if you have been writing in your notebook, if you have recorded it in detail, you will be able to access your imaginary whenever you want. Everything that is recorded is better anchored in our minds, but also, if you forget, you can read it again as many times as you want.

When we clearly know the things we like and what turns us on, remembering them will stimulate our desire whenever we want. So read erotica, watch erotica, listen to erotica, and create your own fantasies. As many as you can. There may be no aphrodisiac foods, but erotic fantasies are infinite: the brain is the most powerful aphrodisiac there is.

THE MOST POWERFUL APHRODISIAC THAT EXISTS IS YOUR OWN BRAIN.

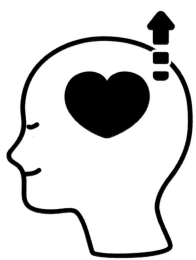

Feel Sexy

Starting to think more about sex, recalling your sensual memory, consuming erotic content and writing down your fantasies will automatically make you feel sexier.

Haven't you noticed that already?

But, even if we increase our volume of fantasies, they don't take up our whole day, and slowly, our hectic lives tend to bring us back to the starting point. How do we avoid this? Well, the same way we remember important appointments: by writing them down or creating reminders that make us think about them again.

Here are a few ideas:

⊖ Clothing and accessories. Wear something that makes you feel sexy or reminds you of a fantasy: a special perfume, lingerie, a fake tattoo, a tie....

⊖ Decoration. Place something in your home that reminds you of something sexual. A picture of a place where you had sex, a sensual figure, handcuffs....

⊖ Allow yourself to be authentic and flamboyant. Say what you think and how you feel.

Act Super Sexy

When I say this, it always creates a little shock amongst you.

"But don't you always say you have to be authentic?"

"What? Aren't you the feminist ranting about gender clichés?"

Yes! It's me. And I insist that clichés are fiction, they are not real. But so are cinema and theater and they can be wonderful. Besides, it's very different to have a cliché imposed on me than it is for me to choose to interpret it.

I don't like cars. I hate driving, and I wouldn't even look at a car catalog with one eye closed. But Girl, I see an Audi ad and it makes me want to drive the whole of Route 66. They sell their product so well that even I, who doesn't care for vehicles, likes it. Well, that's what it's all about. Advertise how sexy you are, but it's not about doing so for others: do it for yourself.

It's not going to be something new to you. It isn't. We all act like that when we fall in love: we go out of our way to seduce. To advertise ourselves. When you just begin to date someone, you always show your best self (or what you think is your best) to impress and attract the attention of your object of desire. You put on your best clothes, the coolest accessory... How long did it take you to dress up for a date? And why don't you do it anymore?

Act sexy! It's not about being dressed up or acting like Marilyn Monroe all day, but giving yourself a publicity moment once in a while.

Write in your notebook which ideas you can come up with to act sexier. One idea is to think about what made you feel sexy when you first got into a relationship. Write it down. And put it into action.

Seduce Yourself, And You Will Seduce the World

A seductive person is one who conveys that she is interested in you and makes you feel special when she is with you. In that way, she generates positive emotions and makes you want to be with her. Seductive people are not the most beautiful or the most intelligent, but they are the ones who make you feel better when they are around.

Seduction is often perceived with a negative connotation, like deception or deceit. But it is not like that at all. Seduction is not cheating. It's about showing your best, showing interest, collaborating and making others feel good. What is so negative about that?

Do you know a seductive person? Think about what they are like and why you consider them seductive. Write it down in your notebook.

There are people who seem to come with the seduction kit as standard, who are born seductresses. Others, however, no matter what they do, can't get anyone's attention. Is being seductive innate? YES! But it is innate for everyone: we are all born seductresses. And there is nothing more seductive than a baby. It's their way of getting milk and kisses, and being in their mother's arms. At some point in your life you have been a baby, and therefore you have been seductive, and surely after that you've been seductive on more than one occasion, although you may have forgotten about it for some reason. How about remembering it?

TIPS to SEDUCE:

- Be authentic and convey what you feel.
- Always look into people's eyes.
- Smile. Joy is transmitted and attracts all eyes.
- Convey warmth and positive messages.
- Listen actively to other people.
- Make the most of your strengths: publicize yourself.
- Always have fun.

When we want to establish a relationship with someone, we instinctively set all our seduction strategies into motion. But when we have succeeded, or have been with that person for a while, many of us stop doing it. Do you think this is true for you?

Think about the last time you acted seductively with someone and why. What did you do? Write it down in your notebook, because I am going to suggest we play a game. For one day, put all those strategies into motion, but to seduce yourself. Pay attention to yourself, listen to what you want, and do it. Look in the mirror and praise what you see.

And the next day, if you feel like it, do it with others.

Love Your Body

In Chapter 2 we made the importance of loving oneself clear. Remember the example of the oxygen mask on the plane? No one is useful to others if they don't take care of themselves first. I recommended you love yourself as much as you love your best friend, as much as the person you love the most, because, in fact, that person should always be you, the one who will be by your side every day of your life.

LOVE YOURSELF AS YOU WOULD LOVE YOUR BEST FRIEND

And what do we do when we love somebody?

- We look at them all the time.
- We are attentive to their desires.
- We take care of them.
- We try to make them feel good.
- We support their health.
- We help them get what they want.

Do you do that with yourself? I hope that after having read Chapter 2 your answer is a big Yes! And if it is not, please take the time to read it again.

From a more erotic point of view, what else do we do when we love somebody?

- You show them your desire.
- You caress them.
- You see to it that they get pleasure.
- You enjoy their pleasure.

Well, it's time for us to talk about doing that with yourself too. To take responsibility for your own pleasure and to show you that you really love yourself.

I LOVE ME

In Chapter 1 we talked about how healthy masturbation is. But masturbation should not be reduced to the pursuit of an orgasm. Autoeroticism should be for genital stimulation and pleasure, but also for stimulation and care of all the other parts of the body, all the senses, self-knowledge and learning.

No two people are alike. We all have different bodies, we come from different contexts, we think differently, and we have had very different histories. That is why there is no one better than you for exploring yourself and learning how you work, how you are and what you like.

I propose you create a ritual of care and self-exploration. What do you think?

Mark it in your calendar, as often as you like, and create it absolutely to your own taste. Vary it, learn about your body and your mind, do your research....

Put into action everything you have discovered in this chapter and everything you discover in the future: create the most aphrodisiac fantasies.

Don't forget:

- A mirror. Look at how beautiful you are and how beautiful your body is. Look at your genitals in detail. Observe the reactions and changes that occur to stimuli and during the sexual response.
- Oils and creams. Pamper your body and genitals with them.
- Aromas. All senses are important in sexual stimulation and smell is not the least. Put scented candles, perfume yourself with something that stimulates your imagination, or add that aroma to the oils and creams you use.
- Toys. As Mae West used to say, sex is like bridge: when you don't have a good partner, it's better to have a good hand. But sometimes the hand gets tired, or doesn't reach certain places. We have wonderful toys that can complement manual tasks.
- Music. Music can transport you to magical places and stimulate all your senses. In the references section I'll include a playlist with music that can accompany you in all your erotic interactions.

"If you want my body and you think I'm sexy
Come on, sugar, let me know If you really need me,
just reach out and touch me
Come on, honey, tell me so"

ROD STEWART: Do Ya Think I'm Sexy?

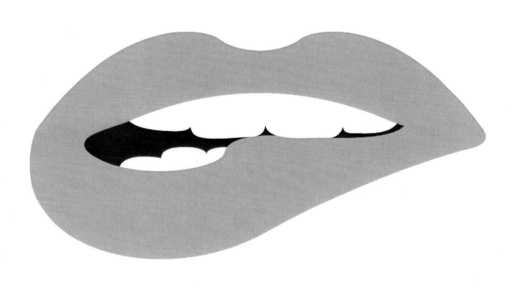

STEP 4: TALKING IS ONLY HUMAN

*"The word asks and is answered
it has wings or goes into tunnels
it detaches itself from the mouth that speaks
and slips through the ear to the eardrum.
The word is so free that it frightens
it divulges secrets without warning
and invents the prayer of atheists
it is the power and it is not the power of the soul
and the spine of the hymns that make a homeland."*

MARIO BENEDETTI: THE WORD

Communication is one of the most developed human skills. It is something that differentiates us from other species: to speak is uniquely human.

People communicate in very different ways, but above all we use ab oral language, written language, or visual, tactile and sonorous symbols. Communicating allows us to express what we think and feel, and thanks to this, we can dialogue, learn and evolve. But everything has a dark side, and communication is as powerful in harming us as it is in helping us, because it also leads us to lie, manipulate and harass. Social media provides a clear example. The Internet and social platforms are a wonderful means of communication that allow us to be informed about almost everything in real time, and to contact millions of people anywhere in the world in an immediate way. Who hasn't looked up an old flirtation on Facebook? Social networks help us find old friends, discover unknown family members, and even find lost pets efficiently and quickly.

But the Internet is just as effective and fast at distributing hoaxes, lies and insults that can even change election results and, worst of all, destroy human lives.

COMMUNICATION CAN BE AS MUCH A WEAPON AS A TOOL

The same thing happens with communication in sexuality and couples: it can cement a lasting relationship, but also destroy it in a few seconds.

"How do you communicate with your partner? Do you think you may have a communication problem?"

When I ask this question in the office, most of you tell me that you don't, that you talk to each other a lot. And I don't doubt that. You probably tell each other everything you've done at work, what's new in the family or the latest gossip you've heard. But ask yourself:

⊖ Do you talk about how you feel about each other?

⊖ Do you express what you think about your relationship?

⊖ Do you always tell each other what you want?

⊖ Do you talk the same way now as you did at the beginning of your relationship?

I am going to give you a few tips that may help you improve your communication.

Talk

We can communicate in many ways, but the best way to clearly share your desires, your fears, your likes and dislikes is: talking.

"Yes, Myriam, but we already know each other so well that we don't need to talk to each other."

I don't doubt it. I'm sure that many of you who are reading this know each other very well and love each other twice as much, but, although sometimes it may seem so, I can assure you that love has not yet caused anyone to acquire superpowers.

LOVE DOES NOT PRODUCE TELEPATHY

No, you can't guess what your partner is thinking, nor can your partner guess what you are thinking. When we believe that because of love we are able to read others' thoughts, that's when reproaches arise:

She knows me perfectly well but does not consider what I want.

She always repeats the same things and she knows I don't like them.

At this point, he/she already should think about what I need first.

It rings a bell, doesn't it?

Well, I'll tell you again so you don't forget it:

LOVE DOES NOT GRANT US SUPERPOWERS

Nor does it give us the best memory in the world, if we didn't already have it. No matter how much you love each other, no matter how close you are, you can only know what the other loves, and how much he/she loves you, if you tell each other and remind each other of it from time to time.

At the hospital cafeteria, they know I like my coffee strong, with oat milk. But the first day I ordered it they didn't know that, and I explained it to them as they were making it.

"No, stronger. Yes, with cold milk. Oat milk, oat milk. Not soy milk, not oatmeal. No, no sugar. No saccharin either. Nothing else. Thank you."

The second day I explained it again the same way.

On the third day, Sonia prepared it for me directly when she saw me coming in, but not without asking me first:

"Your oatmeal brownie, Myriam?"

Most days I nod smiling, but some days I tell her:

"No, thank you, Sonia. Today I'd prefer a green tea."

It's the same with sex. No one can guess what kind of coffee you like if you don't explain it to them in detail. And even if they learn how to prepare your favorite coffee better than you do, you don't always feel like coffee. And if you don't feel like it, you have to say so, and ask for a green tea. Or whatever. Don't forget.

I recommend you find a moment each day to talk about yourselves, even if it's only for the 15 seconds it takes to ask the other person if he/she is happy and well.

With even this small effort, you will improve communication, energy, intimacy and pleasure, and consequently, you will improve DESIRE.

So look for that moment, cherish it, and repeat it every day.

Be Assertive

Assertiveness is a way of communicating in which you are able to freely express your opinions, feelings and opinions, without negatively affecting anyone. To be assertive is to combine firmness and empathy when expressing yourself; to be honest while being respectful and kind.

I love Michael Jackson's music and choreography. I have seen This is it, the documentary that shows the rehearsals of the big tour he was going to do in 2009 and was cut short after his death, many times. I recommend it, it is spectacular. But there is one thing that always strikes me, and that is the assertiveness of its entire cast.

There's a scene where Michael winces and touches his ears.

"Wait a minute, I have to tell you something: I'm trying to listen to myself, but it feels like a fist is being shoved in my ear. I'm having a hard time. I know you don't mean any harm, but it's very difficult for me to work like this."

The music director replies:

"I'm sorry, Michael, is there anything we can change in your headphones to make it work better for you in terms of volume or mix?"

"Maybe if you lowered the volume?"

"Okay, we'll turn it down. Is there anything else you need?"

"No."

"Well, if you see anything else we can do, don't hesitate to let us know."

"Sure, thanks."

Michael Jackson is one of the biggest stars in musical history. At the time he was under brutal pressure to prepare for the tour, along with the personal demons he must have wrestled with. But I flipped out about the way he spoke. He is absolutely assertive.

I am no star and my pressures are those of every normal human being in the world, but I could perfectly imagine myself having said in his place:

"Oh, fuck, this hurts like hell. What a shitty headset, don't you have better ones?"

This would be an example of aggressive communication, not conducive to anything good, as it would undoubtedly make the other person angry and defensive.

He could also have opted for passive communication.

"Is there something wrong, Myriam? You winced."

"No, no. I'm sorry. It's just that these headphones are new, and I have to adapt. But I'll keep going."

This attitude does not assault my conversation partner as much as the previous one, but it does harm me, and it would make me end up in a bad mood, with an earache and a headache.

Michael and the musical director give us a lesson in assertiveness and good work. He says everything he thinks and how he feels without offending anyone and accepting the solutions offered to him. Assertiveness not only facilitates communication, it also improves the energy between everyone and fills us with good vibes.

And we have to bring that assertiveness, saying everything there is to say but without aggression, to all areas: to work, to friends, to our partner, and above all, to sex. Yes, to sex. Because in intimacy, assertiveness will allow us to express our feelings, interests and desires, in line with our opinions and taste, without feeling bad or hurting anyone. Most sexual problems can be solved simply by good sexual communication.

MOST SEXUAL PROBLEMS CAN BE SOLVED BY TALKING

Why are we not assertive in sex?

- Because of shame and fear of being rejected.
  "What will he/she think of me if I say (or ask for) that?"
- Because of inadequate sex education.
  "I won't say that, because it could spoil everything."
- Ignorance of one's own body.
  "I don't know if I'll like that, so I'd better not do it."

I hope that, at this point in the book, you recognize how wrong these ideas are. But just in case, I repeat the most important sentence in this book:

GOOD SEX IS GOOD FOR YOUR HEALTH

And the goal of good sex is satisfaction and pleasure, so you should not hesitate for a second to ask for everything you want and reject everything you don't feel like. By being assertive, people get to know themselves better and allow themselves to enjoy themselves much more, improving their health and well-being.

And this is when someone always says to me:

"But Myriam, with sex you don't have to talk."

"Of course you can talk! You have to talk! Sex is communication!"

In the first chapter, we already talked about the fact that sexuality encompasses reproduction, pleasure and communication. The reproductive function we share with all other living beings, and pleasure with the other mammals, but eroticism, intimacy and love are totally human. I would say almost divine.

And humans have another ability that sets us apart from other animals: we talk!

Want to learn to be more assertive?

Start small: always express your opinions clearly and calmly, respecting others. Never apologize for saying what you think, nor look for justification for your opinion, nor say it in anger, thinking that the other person should have guessed it. It has already been made clear to us that we are not fortune tellers.

You will be surprised by the results.

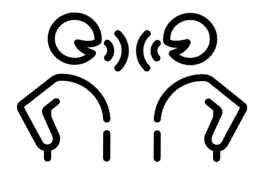

Listen

Communication is not only talking, it is also listening. And just as it has become clear to us that it is essential to speak well, or assertively, we must also listen well: fully attentive, with all our senses focused on the person who transmits his or her message to us.

Listening well is more than just hearing words, it is doing so actively, with empathy and full awareness, without interrupting or judging, and concentrating on the message being transmitted.

When you are listened to, you feel valued and understood; you feel important. Most of the time you don't need opinions or answers: you just need to be heard. A person who is not listened to feels rejected and ignored, and will stop sharing things with the person who has not listened well. That is why it is so important, even if it takes effort.

There is a beautiful example of active listening in the movie Inside Out, when Sadness listens to the Elephant. Here is the link:

https://www.youtube.com/watch?v=t685WM5R6aM

The next time someone you care about wants to tell you something, stop whatever you're doing and listen.

Be Grateful

When we are little, one of the first things we are taught is to ask for things by using "please" and to say "thank you." Thanking someone is not only a sign of politeness, but a sign of appreciation for the good they have done for us.

TO SAY THANK YOU IS TO GIVE RESPECT, LOVE AND VALUE

The moment someone thanks you for something, you usually smile, you feel happy. But science tells us that being thankful is even more beneficial to the person giving thanks, both physically and psychologically. Grateful people tend to be much happier and healthier.

BEING GRATEFUL IMPROVES YOUR HEALTH

It is easy to be grateful for things that strangers do for you. But many times we forget to thank the person closest to us, who is usually the one who deserves it the most.

When was the last time you thanked your partner for something?

Or your mother?

I'd like you to make a gratitude journal. Start it in your notebook and if you like it, decorate a special one just for giving thanks. Each night write down three different things you were grateful for. They can be very simple things: a goodnight kiss, your record collection, the smell of cut grass or the taste of chocolate. You will notice how easily you fill the journal.

It would be wonderful if you kept it all your life, because its benefits are spectacular. Cultivating gratitude allows us to become aware of all the good things we normally take for granted, to focus on the positive and unfocus on the negative.

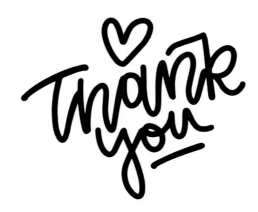

Smile!

Smiling is one of the most present expressions in human beings and although it is modified by learning, it is innate, as can be seen in prenatal ultrasounds, in which babies inside the womb, without having seen anyone smile, smile.

WE SMILE EVEN BEFORE WE ARE BORN

If we were all clear about the benefits of smiling, we would end the day with sore cheeks, as I do every birthday. Smiling is wonderful; when you do it everything seems to get better. And it is true. There are many scientific studies that show that everything improves:

It improves your mood. When you smile, the brain processes that you are happy and releases substances such as serotonin, which bring well-being and improve your mood.

It decreases pain. In addition to serotonin, smiling causes the brain to produce endorphins and other natural painkillers that increase the pain threshold.

It reduces stress. People who smile more often have lower blood levels of adrenaline and cortisol, stress hormones. And if your anxiety is reduced, creativity and productivity increase.

It improves cardiovascular health. Smiling lowers blood pressure and your heart rate.

It boosts your defenses. Both laughter and smiling have been shown to improve the immune system, increasing the number of lymphocytes and non-specific defense proteins such as interferon.

It extends life. There are very curious studies that correlate people who smile more with a 4- to 7-year increase in life expectancy.

It improve your social relationships. It is clear. Smiling not only makes you happy, but also makes others happy. If you smile at a stranger on the street, half the time they will smile back. And those smiles will induce a brain change in those people, improving their day. If you can do that with a stranger, how do you think you would change the lives of the people you love the most?

Kinesthesia is a two-way communication system between your brain and the rest of your body. It is your brain's way of informing itself of changes that have occurred and responding to them.

When you like something, your brain sends the information to the muscles in your face, producing a smile. But the opposite also happens: if you smile, even if you don't want to, your brain begins to secrete substances that improve your mood. And this has been proven.

So, write it down in your notebook:

I AM GOING TO FILL MY DAYS WITH SMILES

But I don't want them to be fake. Although it has been shown that fake smiles can also improve your mood, the feelings generated can be contradictory. It's much better to smile for a reason.

To do this, write a list of things that make you smile and also paste pictures that move you in your notebook.

Tonight when you go to bed, smile, thinking about something on your list. Smile when you wake up tomorrow, smile at people who look at you and see if they smile back. You will be surprised at the results.

Whenever you are feeling down, think of something on your list, and smile. Think about how those smiles have influenced your day and write down your reflections.

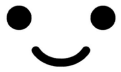

"Let your smile change the world,
but never let the world change your smile."

BOB MARLEY

Respect and Forgive

Most people know what respect is and we desire and demand it, but we do not provide it in the same way to others, and even less to the people who usually deserve it the most, who are the people we live with.

Respecting others is part of the foundation of a healthy social relationship and especially of a couple's relationship. Respect means treating others with the consideration they deserve, accepting their differences and particularities without imposing our own.

NEVER GO TO SLEEP ANGRY WITH YOUR PARTNER

Do you know this popular saying? I have heard it from more than one person. They have all told me that they have heard it from their mothers, their grandmothers, a teacher. It is possible that it derives from a passage in the Bible (Ephesians 4:26-27) that says "Let not the sun go down on your wrath."

Although popular wisdom is not always true (nor is the Bible), this recommendation is more than reasonable and has a neuroscientific justification. During sleep, we process the information we have received during the day and we store it in the brain. Thus, although you may forget the situation that has provoked a negative emotion when you wake up, the emotion that was created remains stored and is also associated with the person who has provoked it. Little by little, this damages the relationship with that person.

So always try to resolve all conflicts before going to sleep.

Write the saying down in your notebook, or better, a more positive affirmation such as:

I ALWAYS RESOLVE MY CONFLICTS

BEFORE I GO TO SLEEP

And highlight it!

Commit!

When we talked about desire, we said that conscious love, rational love was built every day; sharing pleasure, intimacy and emotions with commitment and dedication.

And what is commitment?

Commitment is the willingness of people in a relationship to adapt and fight for a common project. There are as many types of people and couples as there are types of commitment, but whatever they are, they must always be defined and, above all, maintained.

And why is commitment so important?

Because sharing a goal with respect and loyalty brings security, trust and stability to the people who are committed. And this is incompatible with anxiety and fear, thus promoting not only a healthy relationship but also good health.

So I have to get married?

It is not necessary to get married to establish a commitment as a couple. Weddings are social and legal contracts that facilitate a commitment and allow you to make it public. But you can commit in many ways, as long as you establish criteria for your common goal and expectations. These criteria may be quite different from those of other couples. The important thing is to define them clearly and, above all, to respect them.

In your notebook, write down a list of the criteria for commitment that you have or would like to have as a couple. Reflect on the importance you attach to them, whether you could do without them, or whether you would like to change them in some way.

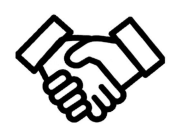

STEP 5: TAKE ME ON A DATE

*"Take me on a date,
let's go to the park,
enter my life unannounced.
Open the door and close your eyes,
Let's gaze at each other, bit by bit.
Give me your hands, feel mine,
like two blind (lovers), St. Lucia..."*

MIGUEL RÍOS: Santa Lucía

I remember the first time I went on a date. I was 17 years old and we had arranged to meet in the afternoon for a coffee at El Sol, a bar in the center of Santander. How nervous I was! I had hardly slept. I dressed in the nicest clothes I had, put on my make-up and perfume, and rehearsed a thousand gestures and witty phrases in front of the mirror. I think I spent more than three hours in the bathroom!

And although a lot has happened since then, I still remember the excitement and how beautiful I felt when I entered the bar and saw the expression of the person who was waiting for me. Yes, I was really spectacular, but it wasn't because of the clothes or the make-up, but because of how special I felt and how unique that moment was going to be for me.

Do you remember that excitement? Do you remember how you used to prepare for those first dates? Well, that's what this step is all about: recovering the importance of our dates and sexual encounters. Because over time, we sacrifice it to other things that occupy our day and our mind.

"I know, but I have other responsibilities now, Myriam."

I don't doubt that. But your health is also important, and that's what we're talking about, remember? Besides, you can do it all.

"Everything? I'll stress myself out, and that decreases desire too."

Not if you do it right. Remember what we talked about in Step Two? If we want to get a lot done, being productive and not getting stressed along the way is crucial....

"Get organized!"

That's right! And to get organized, the first task is to have an agenda. Put sex in your schedule. Make it a date!

Make a Date for Pleasure

When I recommend making a date for sex, something I do quite often in my practice, people look at me with amazement.

"But Myriam, isn't routine supposed to be a relationship killer?"

Well, it depends on what we're talking about. Most people see routine and consistency as boring and negative. But I don't agree with that at all. In fact, I think it's actually the opposite. Routines and habits are the best way to grow, evolve and succeed in life. They are the real key to success. The poor word "routine" is misunderstood and confused with another word, the one that really is a killer, the one that kills desires, fantasies and desires. The real killer is not routine: it's boredom.

ROUTINE DOESN'T KILL PASSION; BOREDOM DOES.

So change your mind and start believing that when it comes to sex, routines and habits are just as good as they are for sports, beauty, study and work. In fact, most enduring couples, those who have been together for many years and are happy, have an established day for sex, even if it is not verbalized.

So, start thinking about a day and time for sex - or do you already have one?

"But Myriam! Without spontaneity isn't it a bit cold?"

Not at all! On the contrary. And I'll give you a good example: food.

Eating is a vital necessity, we have to do it to survive. However, when we feel the impulse of hunger, we don't jump at the first edible thing we see. A lion might do that, but I don't jump and bite a cow if I get hungry while walking in the countryside. Nor do I eat the grass in the meadow, to give a more vegan-friendly example. No way. People usually set a schedule for meals and, in addition, we anticipate and prepare for them: we think about the menu, buy the food, cook it and share it at the table. And not only that; we celebrate special days with much more elaborate meals and set-ups.

What do we do when we have a special dinner at home? Most of us clean and tidy up the house a bit (at least where the guests are going to be), decorate the table, put out our best tablecloth and tableware, prepare or order a special menu... I don't know about you, but I enjoy this from the very first moment I start to organize or prepare for the dinner. The decor, the preparation, the company, the moment? Everything is richer and more exciting when it is done at a special table.

The same thing happens with sex. When you prepare for it with care, when you anticipate and enhance it, sensations are intensified and satisfaction is greater. And although snacking between meals with some chocolate or potato chips can be wonderful, it would never be if that was all you ate.

Take a look at these four options and tell me which meal plan you would enjoy the most:

- I'm walking through the countryside, I'm hungry and I eat some grass and two little flowers.
- It's lunchtime and I have a nice salad that I bring from home in a lunch box, as I do every day.
- I have a date for a few beers in a tapas bar.
- I have been invited to a gastronomic experience at the restaurant of a very creative chef whom I admire very much. I have eaten very little today, so that I can enjoy it more.

Which plan would you choose first, and how would you rank the rest of the options?

If we go by the received wisdom that sex must be spontaneous and "not cold", the top choice would be to eat the grass, right?

But be honest, gastronomically speaking, which meal would you put in your Instagram Reel?

Set Aside Time for Intimacy

One common reason to explain a loss of desire and decreased frequency of sex is lack of time. And it's not just an excuse: lack of time is real. Life is filled with tasks, responsibilities and commitments, and we always end up leaving sex for last. And leaving it for the end is only if we are lucky, because it usually becomes a "well, maybe later", and then there's usually neither time nor desire because we are overcome by sleep and fatigue and everything starts to feel like an uphill battle. Sound familiar?

Did you know that, according to a 2008 Pennsylvania State University study, the IDEAL average time for satisfactory sexual intercourse ranges from 7 to 13 minutes?

And did you know that, according to a HootSuite study, the Spanish population spends an average of 2 hours a day on social media and 3 hours watching TV?

You don't have time for 10 minutes of sex but you spend 2 hours watching Reels? No criticism, of course you have to choose what you want to do, but review the chapter of All You Need is Love and really think about what your priorities are. Laughing at Reels is great fun, but maybe you don't need to spend so much time on them.

If you really want to rekindle your desire and enhance your sexual interactions, you need to start giving them the importance they deserve. And if you care enough to be reading this book, you shouldn't rank it last.

MAKE YOUR HEALTH IMPORTANT: MAKE SEX IMPORTANT

When You're Having Sex, Have Sex!

There's a BMW commercial that I love for what it says. You can see it here:

https://www.youtube.com/watch?v=z-XwiZzKeSg

Since I don't think it has an English version, I'll transcribe the script for you:

"When you're working, work. When you're resting, rest. When you're pedaling, pedal. When you're dancing, dance. When you're jumping, jump. And when you're shouting, shout! If you have to fight, fight. But when you're helping, help. And when you try, try for real. When you advance,

advance. When you play, play. And when you dream, dream. When you win, win. And when you lose, especially when you lose, lose. When you drive, drive."

Paying attention to what you do is the secret to almost everything: efficiency, health, happiness, time management and, of course, the quality of sex.

TO BE, YOU HAVE TO SHOW UP

I have not been able to find out whose phrase this is. But I think it's great: to be, you have to show up. Because if you don't, you are not even there. If you decide to enjoy sex, whether as a couple or not, and you're also looking at your cell phone, the TV, thinking of your worries, your to do list... you're not really present: you're your autopilot, and it will prevent you from enjoying it. And no, no matter how much you joke about women being able to do many things at once and men not, it's a lie. Numerous studies show that multitasking is not a matter of gender and is anything but healthy.

So disconnect from all that noise that prevents you from paying attention and dedicate yourself 100% to prepare an erotic experience free from all distractions.

Surely you're familiar with the concept of Mindfulness. This practice has become very popular in recent years, although meditation based on mindfulness is more than two millennia old.

Mindfulness is based on being aware of the present moment, with acceptance, with curiosity, but without judgment, simply being in the here and now. Being present. It seems easy, but it isn't, because the mind likes to run wild and jump from one place to another. Concentrating takes effort, but if you can manage it, you achieve the greatest peace of mind.

Mindfulness has proven useful in the management of stress and many diseases such as depression and cardiovascular disease.

At the sexual level, there is already talk of Sexfulness, a technique derived from Mindfulness, for sex with full attention, without focusing on objectives or goals, but simply on the present moment and sensations. It is about the journey, not the destination.

Sexfulness proposes a step-by-step enjoyment of sex, creating a balance between mind, emotions and body, leaving everything else aside. In this way it allows you to connect with your partner and full pleasure on a deeper and more complete level.

Key ideas:

⊖ Don't set goals – forget about orgasms, ejaculations or squirts.

⊖ Focus on enjoying the present moment, on enjoying every caress, every word, every kiss. Live here and now.

⊖ Don't act against your desires. Listen to your body and your reactions. Maybe you just feel like caresses. Or maybe nothing at all. Follow your body's desires in the present moment.

⊖ Accept your thoughts and don't blame yourself if they distract you, but release them to become conscious in the present again.

Becoming Gourmet

According to the Cambridge Dictionary, a gourmet is defined as "a person who knows a lot about food and cooking, and who enjoys eating high-quality food." We also usually call everything that is characterized by quality and sophistication "gourmet". There are people who are little gourmets from the cradle, but in general, becoming gourmet is a skill you can learn. Like everything!

I have always loved cheese. That's why, the day that Piedad, one of my choir mates, invited all the choir members to a cheese tasting, I was thrilled to sign up. Piedad is the world's greatest expert in Mahón cheese (as my friend Antonia from Mallorca is for sobrasada). I knew I was going to enjoy this experience.

"Girls, we will meet at the Binifadet winery, where we will have a cheese and wine tasting."

Wine? I didn't like that so much. I had signed up for the cheese. Wine never appealed to me. I didn't understand wine at all, and when it came to choosing one at a restaurant, I would always throw the menu into someone else's hands as if it were burning. No, I would not drink wine.

But Piedad explains everything so well and so beautifully that I ended up trying the wine. And in every sip and in every bite of cheese, I looked for everything she told us to look for: blueberries, currants, wood, leather... It was an incredible experience. From that day on, I not only appreciate and enjoy a glass of wine, but I have learned to look for new sensations in each and every mouthful I taste: textures, smells, memories, emotions... Piedad made me become a little bit of a wine aficionado.

If you have the chance to experience a tasting, don't think twice: it is a wonderful experience. But you can start experimenting with being a gourmet at home today.

When you have lunch or dinner, turn off all screens and concentrate only on what you are doing. Savor every bite and every sip, find all the flavors, aromas and textures. Also notice how it leaves your mouth, how it makes you feel, what happens in your body before, during and after. Eat and drink slowly; pay attention to everything. You will discover things you never noticed before. Write all your findings and sensations in your notebook.

"Very nice, Myriam. But what does this have to do with sex?"

Well, everything! Absolutely everything. Because what I'm suggesting you do will stimulate and sharpen all your senses, so much so that it will increase your gastronomic pleasure infinitely. And the same, exactly the same, can be achieved in sex: having gourmet sex that exponentially increases your sexual pleasure.

"Gourmet sex?"

Yes, gourmet, because it is about enjoying quality sex, using all your senses, paying attention and enjoying the whole process. At the tasting, the pleasure was in feeling the wine, not in drinking down the whole glass. I enjoyed Piedad's tasting very much, but only the process, not the purpose. I didn't want it to end, I wanted to keep tasting those flavors. Gourmet sex should be the same. Having an orgasm is not the goal. Neither is ejaculating. The purpose, the goal, is to set all the senses in motion and concentrate on enjoying them.

REMEMBER THAT THE JOURNEY IS THE GOAL

I've told you this before. And so it is. The secret of good sex is not a map of destinations with all the letters of the alphabet on them, nor a catalog of positions and toys. That's all fine and dandy, but the key is to pay attention to your feelings and emotions, to recognize them, to enjoy them and let them grow without fear or shame, without thinking about yesterday or tomorrow, only in the now and to the maximum.

In great anxiety and stress a phenomenon called "tunnel vision" occurs. In these circumstances the perception is altered so that you only see a part of things, as if you were seeing the world from a tunnel or through a small hole in the wall. The cause of this phenomenon is adrenaline, and its purpose is to focus our attention on the danger that is supposedly causing anxiety, so we can defend ourselves or flee from it. This can be very useful if you're running from a lion, but is not so useful when the cause is stress, or a bad working relationship, because the loss of our 360-degree vision prevents us from seeing a solution to our problem that we might have beyond the tunnel. We only focus on one thing, the one that is in our tunnel and we forget about everything else.

This is how sex has been seen in our society, either by seeing it as negative, or by focusing only on intercourse and penetration with the penis. Maybe talking about sex causes a lot of stress to some people, but I assure you that this anguish would disappear if we broke the wall surrounding the tunnel and saw sex as it is, free of fears and myths, from 360 degrees, and enjoyed all our senses, our whole bodies, and especially the most important sexual organ we have: the brain.

Not All Pleasure is Sexual

I hope that you have already made your date with pleasure. And I hope it has become clear to you that not all sex is about having an orgasm or genitalia. I would also like to add that not all intimacy as a couple on these dates needs to be about sex. It is very important, and also very enriching, to make room for moments of intimacy without a sexual objective, such as hugging, caressing, relaxing for a while together, and doing activities that you both enjoy.

Open your notebook and write down what "non-sexual" things you would like to do with your partner.

Here are some examples:

- Cuddling while watching a movie you both love.
- Dancing to a slow song that means something to you.
- Taking a nap without any clothes on.
- Massaging your feet with aromatic oils.
- Having a head massage.
- Watching a comedy or telling each other jokes: laughing is wonderful.
- Going to an amusement park and riding the roller coaster together.

Θ Having a gourmet tasting!

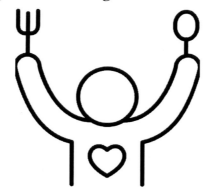

STEP 6: BREAK THE RULES

*"Everybody break it
Every rule every constriction
My papa told me to be home by now
But my party has just begun
Maybe he'll understand that I got to be
To be the freak that God made me
So many things that I want to try
Got to do them before I die
This is my sexual revolution"*

MACY GRAY: Sexual Revolution

I like technology. Although I was born and raised in the paper era, I have adapted quite well to our technological evolution, and I enjoy trying out all kinds of apps and gadgets. That doesn't stop me from occasionally going into panic mode when my computer decides to crash and stop working, usually at the worst possible moment. Fortunately, for these crises there is always the first law of computer repair, the one we all know: the reboot.

The reboot is like a magic spell. You turn everything off, turn it back on, and suddenly everything works as if nothing had ever happened. You've probably restarted your computer or your mobile phone more than once when they crashed, right? And do you know why that happens? Do you know what the magic trick is? It's easy: by restarting, we eliminate all the superfluous and dispensable things that get in the way and prevent us from doing what's really important.

When the superfluous disappears from the scene, everything flows and works again. That is exactly what I would like you to learn to do in this step: reset yourself.

REBOOT

To do this, the first thing you have to do is become aware of the moments and situations in which you get blocked and get stuck -- like that computer. The next time you don't feel well: stop, reflect, investigate and detect what is holding you back and hurting you.

STOP AND OBSERVE YOURSELF

When you suspect what is getting in the way: close it, put it away and remove it.

I would like you to relax for a moment and write in your notebook:

ϴ When was the last time you felt bad about sex, and how were you feeling before that? Describe the situation and how you felt.

ϴ Why do you think you felt that way? With all that you have learned, you may find more than one cause., List them all.

ϴ Analyse all the causes and consider what you can do to eliminate or minimise them. Write down all the possible remedies and make a commitment to do try them.

ϴ Do you think there is anything else you can do to improve the situation?

ϴ Is there something new you would like to try? Write it down. Reflect, analyse, break your old rules and try new ideas, but above all, allow yourself the luxury of being wrong, forgiving yourself and laughing at your mistakes.

*"If you want different results,
do not do the same things".*

ALBERT EINSTEIN

Practice smart sex

Sexual intelligence is a person's ability to intelligently and positively manage their sexuality. Sexually intelligent people enjoy all their sexual interactions and help their partners do the same. To do this, they work on their self-awareness, their perception of their environment, their emotions, and their sexual learning.

Being sexually intelligent does not mean that you are more seductive or more beautiful, nor is it something that you are born with. Being sexually intelligent is something you learn every day, and you get better at with practice. And you are already working on it, by reading and practising what I recommend in this book!

Always think critically

Do you know what critical thinking is? It is the ability to analyse and evaluate the information you receive, without anything external intervening and biasing your perception. It is not about judging or condemning, but analysing and verifying, seeing what others may not see and listening to what others do not hear. To think critically is to refuse to accept that something is so simply because it has always been the case, or because someone you know has asserted it. It is thinking for yourself and choosing what is best for you, not what pleases someone else.

Please always think critically and for the good of humanity, but when it comes to sex, think even more critically: sexuality is riddled with myths and falsehoods.

Be curious

Curiosity is the key to intelligence. Curious people tend to be smarter, because without curiosity, there is no motivation. And without motivation, there is no direction and no goals. If you have reached this page, you are interested in the subject, so don't stop!

Don't finish when you've come to the conclusion of this book! On the internet there is wonderful and fun information about sex and desire. At the end of the book I leave you a few references that I love. But every day there are new ones. Learn! Discover! Innovate!

Try new things!

Don't hesitate! Experiment! Try anything you feel like, as long as it's safe, consensual and doesn't cause harm. Come on, get out of your comfort zone now! In addition to this book, I've published a book of ideas for couples and I'd love you to download it. It's called 111 'sexideas' for couples. As an appetizer, here is a few of them:

Write down your sexual fantasies

And ask your partner to write down his or her fantasies too. Fantasies are thoughts that eroticise the mind and are only meant to arouse and increase desire. Everyone has their own sexual fantasies, and they can either be consciously created or appear spontaneously.

Write them down and read them. You can rate them, compete and perhaps put them into practice.

Try sexting your partner

Sexting consists of sending erotic messages over the internet or smartphone. You can do it with photos, video, audio or text messages, but they should always be racy. Remember to do it safely, and it's preferable if you are not recognisable in them.

The expectation created by good sexting can be the best aphrodisiac for an unforgettable encounter.

Tie me up!

To immobilise or being immobilised can be very exciting and erotic. The literary trilogy by E. L. James and the influence of her Mr. Grey made submission and domination games trendy, as along with the acronym BDSM. The acronym is derived from the words Bondage, Domination, Discipline, Submission, Sadism and Masochism. It includes a wide variety of sexual practices, but it is also a philosophy and a way of life.

You may love the whole world of BDSM or you may just be turned on by its sensual aesthetics. Either way, treat it with respect and enjoy it safely, sensibly and consensually.

Get back to petting

Remember your teenage years and your first sexual encounters? It was all rubbing, touching, kissing and caressing in a corner at school or on a park bench. Well, that's what petting is: kissing, caressing, touching and nothing more. Or nothing less.

How about going back to those years? Go back to having sex without taking your clothes off, without penetration and without focusing on orgasm, just enjoying an unhurried and erotic sexual encounter with all your senses. And you can even go back to the park!

Let's play!

Playing is wonderful. There is nothing more human than playing and toys. Erotic toys are perfect for incorporating something different into your relationship and for your self-knowledge sessions. There are all kinds: dildos, vibrators, suckers, remote-controlled, synchronised, rings, plugs, balls .... Sex toys give pleasure, create fun, enhance and heal. So a good sex idea is to go with your partner to a sex shop or visit a specialised online shop together.

Try edging

Edging is a sexual practice based on stopping just before reaching orgasm, and then restarting the stimulation. This maintains a very high level of sexual arousal for as long as possible, which means that when the orgasm is released it is much more intense and prolonged.

Eat me!

"Sploshing" consists of smearing or being smeared. Just doing it on your naked body is exciting enough, but if you do it with something you love to eat, it can be extraordinary. Can you imagine what it would be like with chocolate or your favourite ice-cream?

Talk Dirty

Dirty talk is nothing more than saying "dirty things" to each other. Talking dirty in the ear, avoiding terms that may be offensive to your partner, can be very exciting. Lose your fear of dirty talk; you may be surprised at how stimulating and provocative it is. Tell your partner what you like about him or her, what you want to do or have her/him do to you, describe what you are doing, and how it makes you feel.

Explore tantric sex

Tantric sex is a practice surrounded by myths that generates a lot of curiosity among couples. It is based on tantra, a thousand-year-old eastern philosophy that focuses on the sexual energy of the individual to reach ecstasy. Tantric sex has more and more fans, and its aim is to enjoy sex in a fuller and more tranquil way, without focusing on the genitals or orgasm, but on the whole body and mind.

Do you feel like trying any of these ideas with your partner?

Don't hesitate! Try it, and don't be afraid of mistakes. At the end of our lives, people have more regrets about what they haven't done than about our mistakes. If you mess up, if you don't get it right, if it doesn't work out in the end, there is nothing better in life than a good laugh and I assure you that you will have a funny story to tell.

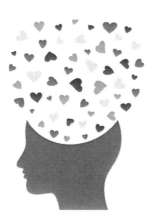

STEP 7: YOUR OWN STEP

"Nobody can tell you
There's only one song worth singing
They may try and sell you
Cause it hangs them up
To see someone like you
But you gotta make your own kind of music
Sing your own special song
Make your own kind of music
Even if nobody else sings along"

CASS ELLIOT: Make your own kind of music

We are all different, all of us. There is not one person on the face of the Earth exactly the same as another.

"Excuse me Myriam, but what about identical twins?"

True, but I assure you that even they are not absolutely the same. Identical twins come from the same egg or zygote, so their genetic make-up is exactly the same. But throughout their life, depending on various environmental factors, the expression of these genes will change, creating differences between them. These are called epigenetic modifications, to which we are all subject, for better and for worse (which is why healthy habits are so important).

So I insist:

WE ARE ALL DIFFERENT

And the fact that everyone is different is something very magical, but it makes it very difficult for us to establish criteria for diagnoses and medical treatments. If all people were exactly the same, we would all have the same symptoms when faced with an illness, and it would be super easy to diagnose and even easier to know the best way to treat it.

But that's not how things work: not everyone has the same symptoms when faced with a problem, and not everyone responds to a treatment in the same way.

Scientific studies and medical statistics help us create diagnostic strategies and effective therapies for the majority of people, but there will always be a percentage of people for whom what is established and statistically effective will not work. And this is something we must always take into account.

That is why we say that medicine is not only a science but also an art. And to be an artist you have to be very open-minded and never forget that each person is wonderfully unique.

I have not forgotten this. And in this book I've summarised the steps I usually follow in my practice and in my workshops. I assure you that most people who report loss of desire get better almost from the very first step. But there will be a few people who need something more: their own approach.

WE ARE ALL DIFFERENT

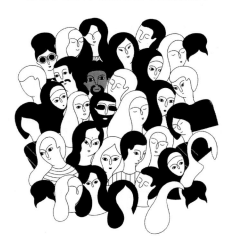

YOU CAN'T MAKE COFFEE FOR EVERYONE: WE DON'T ALL LIKE IT AND IT DOESN'T SUIT EVERYONE.

Check your medical history and your first aid kit

Did you know that there are a lot of diseases and health problems that can affect desire? Not only that, but many of the drugs used to treat them can also affect desire. Sometimes we can't avoid taking them, but knowing that they may be the cause of our loss of desire can help us understand what's wrong and motivate us to intensify the other strategies we've learned can help.

Review your medical history and the package inserts in your medicine cabinet, and see if anything you have or take is on the list:

Here are some of the illnesses that affect desire:

- Stress
- Anxiety and depression
- Diabetes
- Thyroid disease
- Obesity, metabolic syndrome and sleep apnea
- High blood pressure
- Cardiovascular disease
- Cancer, especially breast, genital and prostate cancer
- Neurological diseases
- Rheumatological diseases such as arthritis or fibromyalgia
- Sexual dysfunction
- Gynaecological problems such as endometriosis, climacteric syndrome or menopausal genitourinary syndrome
- Urological problems such as incontinence or prostate hyperplasia

And here are some drugs that can affect desire:

⊖ Antidepressants such as paroxetine and citalopram

⊖ Anxiolytics such as diazepam and alprazolam

⊖ Diuretics such as spironolactone

⊖ Antihypertensives, such as alfamethyldopa and propanolol

⊖ Antiepileptics such as gabapentin and topiramate

⊖ Antihistamines such as diphenhydramine and chlorphenamine

⊖ Gastrointestinal drugs such as omeprazole or cimetidine

⊖ Anovulatory contraceptives

⊖ Antiestrogens such as tamoxifen

⊖ Anti-androgenic drugs such as cyproterone

⊖ Opioids such as morphine, hydrocodone and phenytoin

⊖ Chemotherapy and radiotherapy

Toxins also affect desire and other phases of sexual response:

⊖ Tobacco

⊖ Alcohol

⊖ Heroin and other opiates

⊖ Amphetamines

⊖ Marijuana

⊖ Cannabis

Talk to your doctor

You may have one of the problems I listed. Remember that having the problem addressed, such as diabetes or thyroid disease, can improve your desire. And, of course, even more so if you can treat it, as would be the case with problems related to menopause. That is why it is essential that you consult your doctor, who may also consider changing a drug you are taking for another that has less effect on your desire. If you are abusing any of the toxic substances I listed, it may be time for you to moderate and improve your health and general well-being.

There are also drugs to increase your desire

When I first saw the list of drugs related to sexual dysfunction, my heart dropped. Who doesn't have one of them in their medicine cabinet? Are we all doomed to lose our desire over time? Fortunately not: the drugs on the list are factors that can negatively influence desire, but are not usually the only culprits. However, if you can swap them for something that doesn't affect sexual apetite, so much the better.

But pharmacology can also have a positive effect on desire, and in fact, more and more drugs have been shown to improve libido. Of course, within this group of pro-desire drugs we could consider all those that alleviate the conditions that we have seen to affect desire negatively, for example, all those that treat and improve vaginal dryness, climacteric symptoms, the pain of endometriosis or sexual dysfunction. All of these would improve desire by eliminating some of the factors that make it worse. But more and more drugs and phytopharmaceuticals are becoming available that are specially formulated to directly improve desire. Here are some of them:

ϴ Testosterone: This treatment can improve sexual desire and satisfaction, but is not without side effects.

ϴ DHEA: Dehydroepiandrosterone or DHEA is a hormone produced in the adrenal gland, a precursor of the sex hormones androgens and oestrogens. Its ability to increase testosterone levels appears to be linked to increased libido.

ϴ Flibanserin: This was the first drug approved in the US for loss of desire in women. Its results are modest. It is not approved in Europe.

ϴ Phosphodiesterase inhibitors such as sildenafil: Their main indication is male erectile dysfunction but they also stimulate desire in men and, according to some studies, also in women.

- Bupropion: An antidepressant that may improve desire, arousal and orgasms in premenopausal women.

- Bremelanotide: Appears to increase arousal and desire through increased dopamine. Also not approved in Europe.

- Tribulus terrestris: Medicinal plant that improves desire by increasing testosterone levels.

- Damiana or Turnera diffusa: A shrub native to the Americas, whose leaves are used as a physical and mental tonic and which also improves libido by increasing testosterone.

- Saffron or Crocus sativus: Seems to enhance desire through an increase in serotonin, noradrenaline and dopamine.

- Andean Maca or Lepidium meyenii: Maca is a plant native to Peru, used as a restorative and to improve vitality, desire and sexual vigour.

Consider therapy

Sometimes the loss of desire can be associated with something much deeper, something that has affected you on an emotional level that you may not even remember. Other times, it may be a couple's problem that you haven't been able to resolve with each other. Solving these issues can be your own step. And that's where sexologists come in.

A sexologist is a trained professional who specialises in human sexuality and can carry out various tasks in this field. Sexologists dedicate themselves to sex education, scientific research, information and dissemination, counselling, and to therapeutic intervention in sexual and couple problems – this is what we call sex therapy.

You will probably have improved a lot with these steps, but sometimes it is not enough. Or maybe you have also discovered through these steps that a particular problem needs to be solved. Remember that there are excellent professionals who can help you.

"To find yourself, think for yourself"
SOCRATES

LASTLY

I am very happy to see that you have read the seven steps and are getting to the end of the book. If you are one of those who have been doing the recommendations one by one, step by step, you must have started to notice some changes.

Remember the test you took at the beginning? Check the score you got. I'm pretty sure you will have improved quite a lot, although you will notice it much more as time goes by. Because even though you'll be done with this book in a few pages, I would like you to keep going. I have shown you the seven pillars upon which you can build your desire. You already have the foundation. Now it's up to you to make it taller, bigger, to your liking.

Sexuality has gone from being a taboo subject to being everywhere. A few years ago society denied sex and now it is absolutely hypersexualised. And neither is healthy, because although we are now bombarded with information about sex, most of it is neither true nor based on science.

Never forget that everyone should be able to live and enjoy their sexuality in a safe and autonomous way, without fear or shame and according to how they feel or think. We all have the right to the pleasure we want.

This 7-week apprenticeship is a journey towards desire, but also towards your own evolution and growth. Don't stop here. You have already obtained the first tools to start., Integrate them into your daily life, learn more, and share with me over social media. Don't remain on the ground floor! Build a cathedral or a skyscraper.

PURSUE YOUR DESIRE!

PURSUE YOUR DESIRE!

PURSUE YOUR DESIRE!

"And when I was surrendering to death on the ground, I was awakened by the beating of your wings"

ANGÉLICA RIBES

ABOUT THE AUTHOR

Myriam Ribes

Writer, medical specialist in Obstetrics and Gynaecology, expert in Human Sexuality and Sex Education, and Master in Medical Sexology and Sexual Health.

She works as a gynaecologist and sexologist on the island of Menorca.

myriamribes.com

@myriamribes

Manufactured by Amazon.ca
Acheson, AB